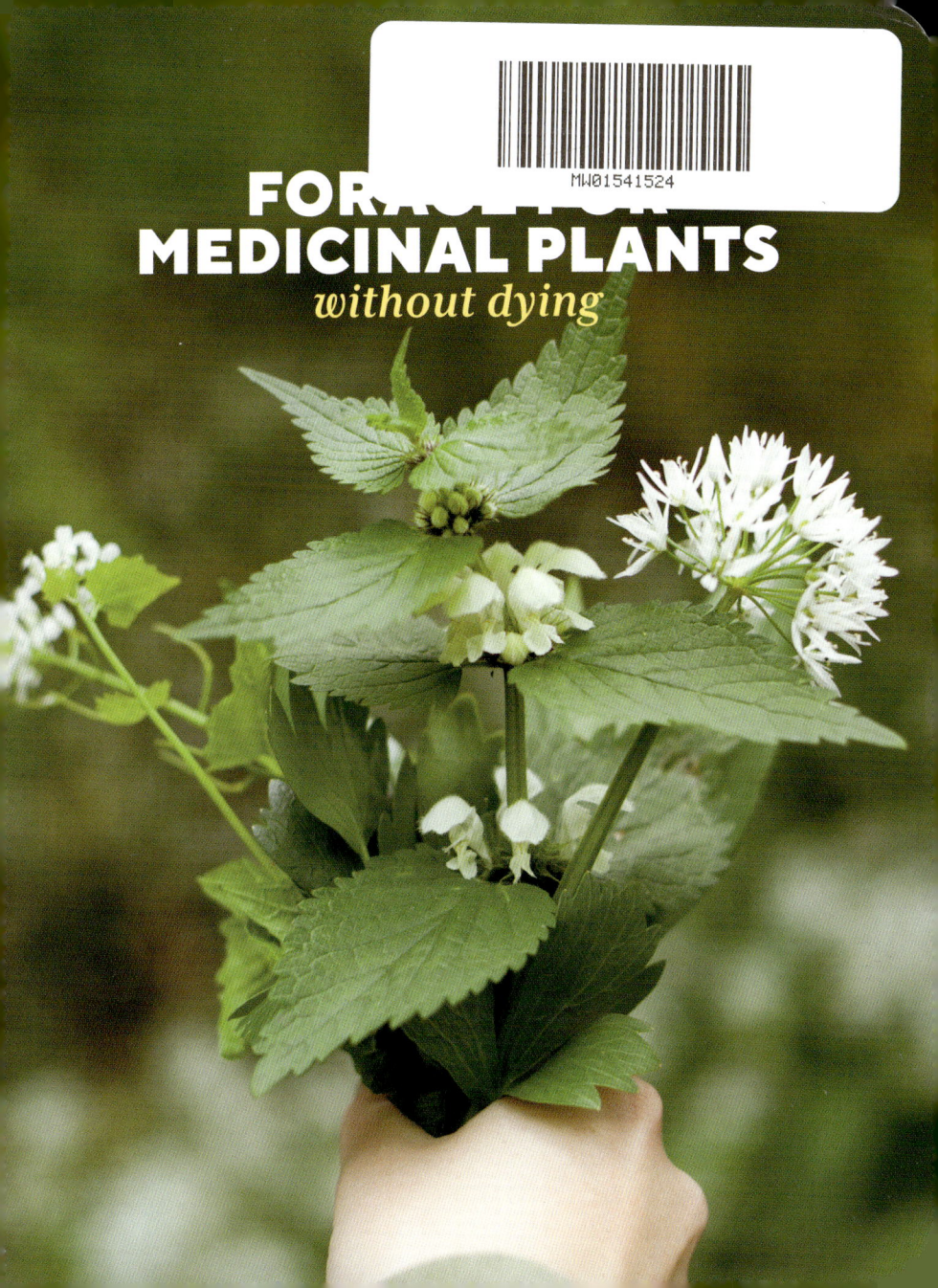

FORAGE FOR MEDICINAL PLANTS
without dying

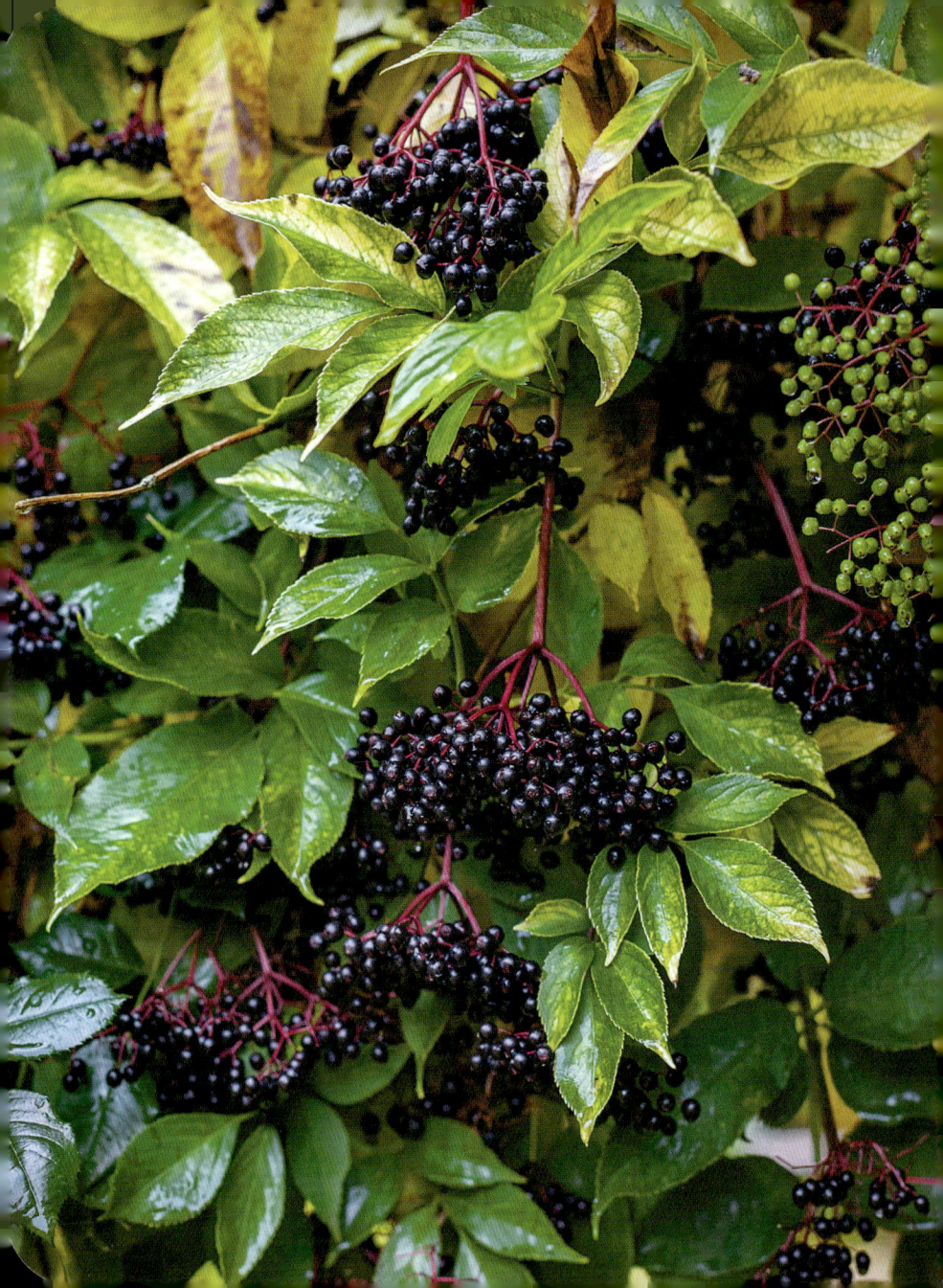

HOW TO FORAGE FOR MEDICINAL PLANTS

without dying

An Absolute Beginner's Guide to
IDENTIFYING 32 HEALING WILD HERBS

BRANDON RUIZ

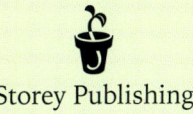

Storey Publishing

The mission of Storey Publishing is to serve our customers by
publishing practical information that encourages
personal independence in harmony with the environment.

Edited by Gwen Hawkes and Carleen Madigan
Art direction and book design by Erin Dawson
Text production by Jennifer Jepson Smith

Cover photography by © alffalff, back 2nd fr. t.; DeOren Robinson, back author; © Hans Verburg, back 2nd fr. b.;
© Maleo/Shutterstock.com, IBC; © Marianne Pfeil/Shutterstock.com, IFC; © nnattalli/Shutterstock
.com, front; © nickkurzenko/iStock.com, back t.; © Wirestock Creators/Shutterstock.com, back b.
Interior photography credits appear on page 255

Text © 2026 by Brandon Ruiz

All rights reserved. Hachette Book Group supports the right to free expression and the value of copyright. The purpose of copyright is to encourage writers and artists to produce the creative works that enrich our culture. The scanning, uploading, and distribution of this book without permission is a theft of the author's intellectual property. If you would like permission to use material from the book (other than for review purposes), please contact permissions@hbgusa.com. Thank you for your support of the author's rights.

The information in this book is true and complete to the best of our knowledge. All recommendations are made without guarantee on the part of the author or Storey Publishing. The author and publisher disclaim any liability in connection with the use of this information.

The publisher is not responsible for websites (or their content) that are not owned by the publisher.

Storey books may be purchased in bulk for business, educational, or promotional use. Special editions or book excerpts can also be created to specification. For details, please contact your local bookseller or the Hachette Book Group Special Markets Department at special.markets@hbgusa.com.

This publication is intended to provide educational information for the reader on the covered subject and is intended only as a resource. Any reader who forages for wild plants and chooses to ingest or use them for any other purposes does so at their own risk; without a 100 percent positive identification, no wild plant should ever be consumed or used in topical or any other preparations. This publication is not intended to take the place of personalized medical counseling, diagnosis, and treatment from a trained health professional. Please consult a physician or other health professional if needed.

Storey Publishing
210 MASS MoCA Way
North Adams, MA 01247
storey.com

Storey Publishing is an imprint of Workman Publishing, a division of Hachette Book Group, Inc., 1290 Avenue of the Americas, New York, NY 10104. The Storey Publishing name and logo are registered trademarks of Hachette Book Group, Inc.

ISBNs: 978-1-63586-949-1 (paperback);
978-1-63586-950-7 (ebook)

Printed in China by R. R. Donnelley on paper from responsible sources
10 9 8 7 6 5 4 3 2 1

APS

Library of Congress Cataloging-in-Publication Data on file

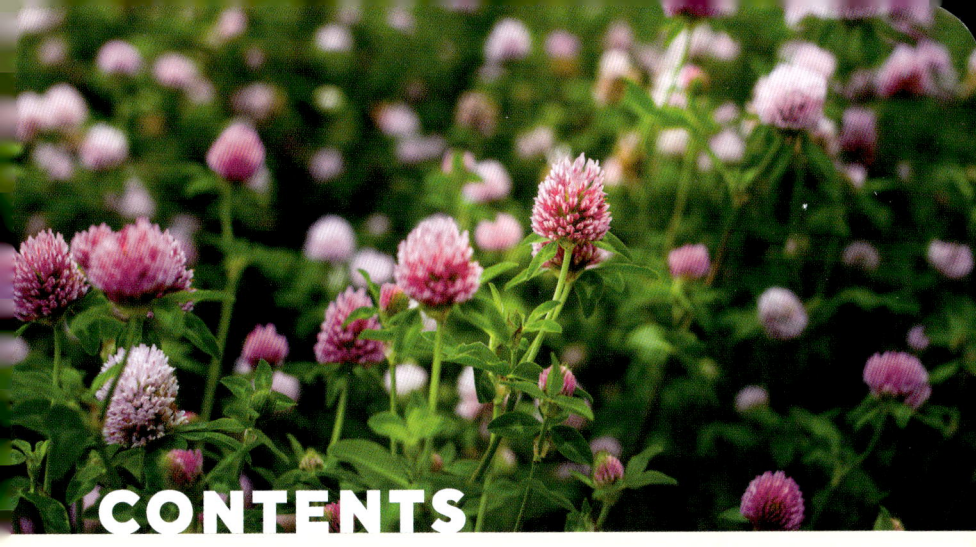

CONTENTS

INTRODUCTION: Why Forage? 8
The Power of Plant Medicine 8
About This Book 11

CHAPTER 1:
RESPONSIBLE FORAGING 15

Ethics in Foraging 16

CHAPTER 2:
HOW TO IDENTIFY A PLANT 25

Combining Traditional and Technical Knowledge 26
The Importance of Proper Identification (i.e., Not Dying) 27
Plant Anatomy 28

CHAPTER 3:
WHAT TO BRING, WHERE TO GO, AND WHEN TO FORAGE 37

Tools for Foraging 38
Where to Forage 41
When to Forage 46
Cleaning and Preserving 48

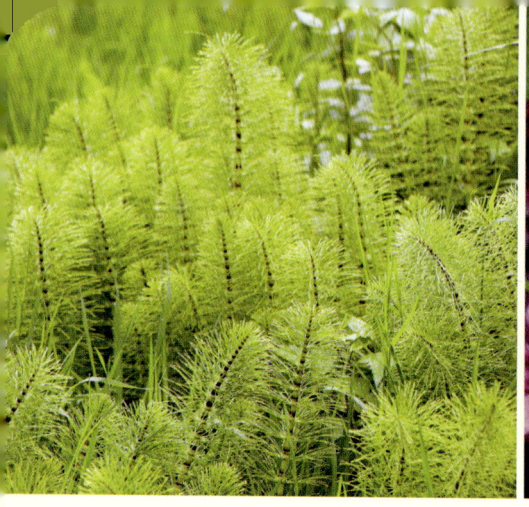
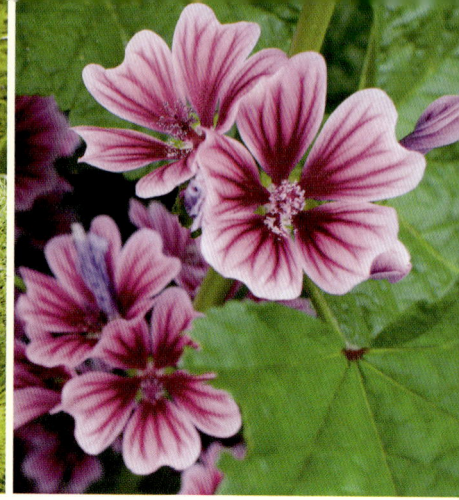

CHAPTER 4:
WONDERFUL WEED MEDICINE 53

Dandelion 54
Cleavers 58
Chickweed 62

Plantain 66
Sweet Annie 70
Garlic Mustard 74

Mugwort 79
Japanese Knotweed 83
Kudzu 87

CHAPTER 5:
WILD HERBS FROM THE FIELD 93

Mullein 95
Violet 98
Burdock 103
Red Clover 106

Wild Lettuce 110
Spanish Needle 114
Yarrow 119
Motherwort 122

Horsetail 126
Wild Rose 130
Elderberry 135
Mallow 141

CHAPTER 6:
FOREST MEDICINE 145

Black Walnut 146
Stinging Nettle 151
Oregon Grape 156
Bee Balm 160

Honeysuckle 164
Raspberry 168
Sumac 172
Mimosa 177

Pine 181
Reishi 185
Linden 190

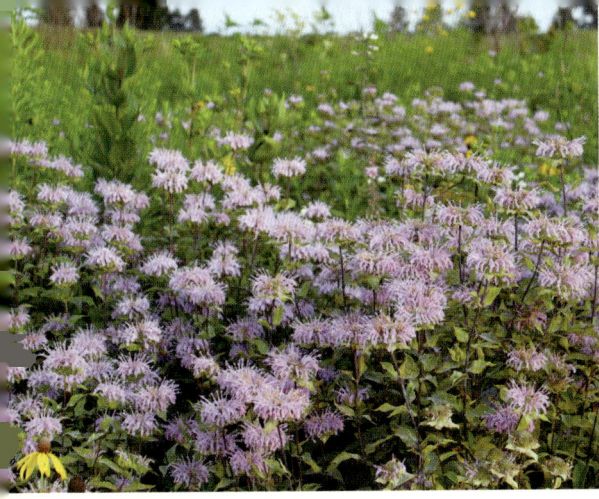
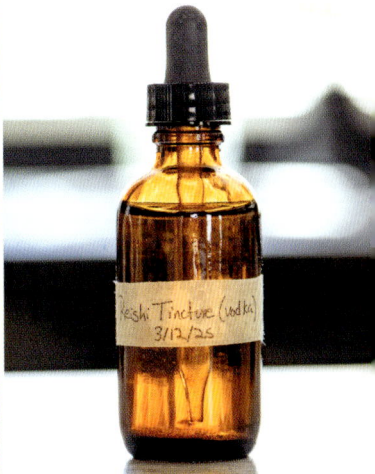

CHAPTER 7:
MAKING MEDICINE 195

Understanding Plant Medicine 196
Making Medicine Safely 196
What You'll Need to Make Herbal Medicine 198

CHAPTER 8:
BASE RECIPES FOR MAKING MEDICINE 205

Infusions 206
Decoctions 212
Tinctures 214
Glycerin Extracts 221
Herbal Vinegars 224
Herbal Steams 226
Topical Medicines 228

CHAPTER 9:
FOOD AS MEDICINE 237

Medicinal Foods 238

Symptom Guide 245
Resources 246
Index 248

INTRODUCTION
Why Forage?

WELCOME TO THE WORLD OF FORAGING! There's a vast and incredible world of plant life growing all around us: in forests, meadows, and our backyards. The plants that we often ignore or overlook can contain powerful healing medicines. This book is a guide to help you see the natural world in a new way, a resource to help you support and heal your body naturally, and an invitation to a more grounded, engaged way of living.

The Power of Plant Medicine

Foraging medicinal plants has changed my life, and the lives of countless others, for the better. When we use plants as medicine, we take our healing into our own hands and gain so much more than just a tea or tincture. We engage in a timeless ancestral experience. Connecting with the natural world and allowing plants to heal us nourishes not only our bodies but our spirits as well. A holistic understanding of health and wellness acknowledges that our well-being is not limited to nutrients, compounds, and calories, but includes our emotional and spiritual health.

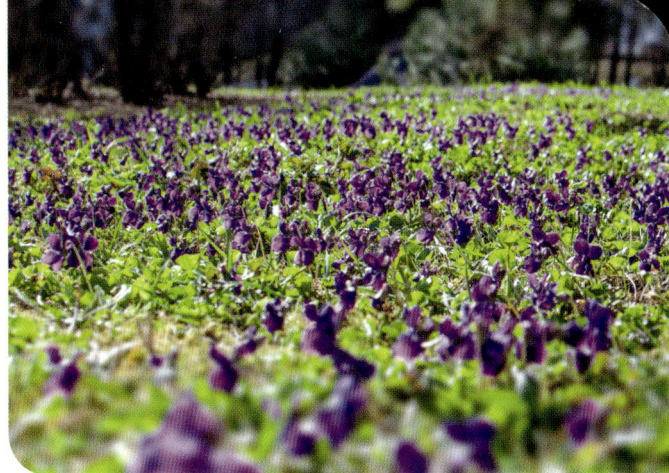

As you start foraging, you'll be surprised by the abundance of medicinal plants growing all around you.

The modern pharmaceutical industry has tempted many people to approach herbal medicine the same way they use pharmaceuticals—looking for a quick fix or a Band-Aid for their health problems. But herbal medicine demands more attention than that. It invites us to slow down, get curious, and consider our well-being from a holistic perspective. How do our lifestyles affect wellness? How are our daily rhythms impacting us? What kind of support and enrichment do we need? Medicinal plants invite us on a journey into our overall wellness.

FORAGING IN COMMUNITY

One of the unique joys and benefits of foraging is the community it creates. Through foraging and working with wild plants, I've gained an enormous network of foragers, herbalists, chefs, and more. You know someone is truly a foraging friend when they happily stop the car to check out a plant spotted 50 feet off the highway or detour completely out of their way to investigate an interesting herb when walking around town. Those are my people—and they can be yours, too!

As you begin working with medicinal plants, you'll discover that one of the best resources for learning is other people. Elders, folks in your neighborhood, or even an online group can all be helpful sources of information. Herbal wisdom is passed from person to person, from generation to generation; as you build your foraging community, you'll build your knowledge.

CONNECTING WITH NATURE

There's certainly nothing wrong with using dried or prepackaged herbs, but when we interact with a living plant, we learn so much more. Being in and connecting with nature is nourishing in a way no supermarket kale can replicate. We can find healing in tending and stewarding plants, not just in consuming them. Our ancestors around the world all understood this.

Plants have personalities, grow differently depending on their environment, and react to seasonal conditions by creating more medicinal compounds, changing colors, and developing new growth patterns. If we don't interact with the living, growing plant, we miss these aspects entirely. Foraging for plants ourselves gives us invaluable insight into the nuances of plant life and how these plants impact our health.

> As you build your foraging community, you'll build your knowledge.

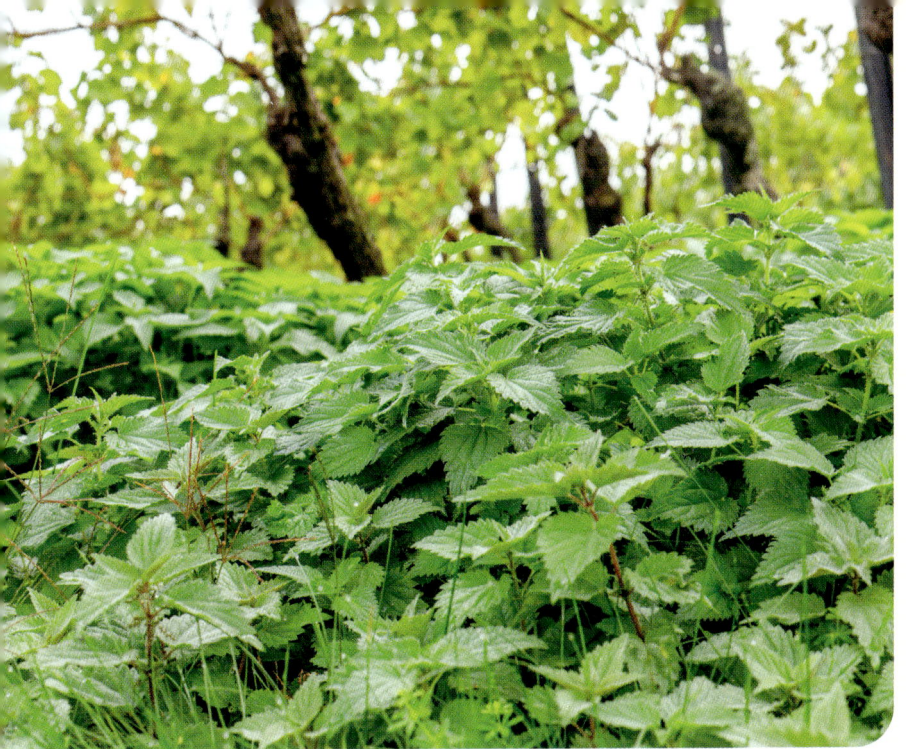

The unique environment in which a plant grows, from the soil to the sun, impacts its medicinal properties. Nettles have been shown to synthesize more bioactive compounds when exposed to drought conditions.

About This Book

The botanical world is vast and complex, but this book is designed to be a beginner-friendly invitation to the art of working with medicinal plants. While these plants may take a lifetime to truly understand, this guide will equip you with the skills to confidently identify, harvest, and use some of the most common and useful varieties.

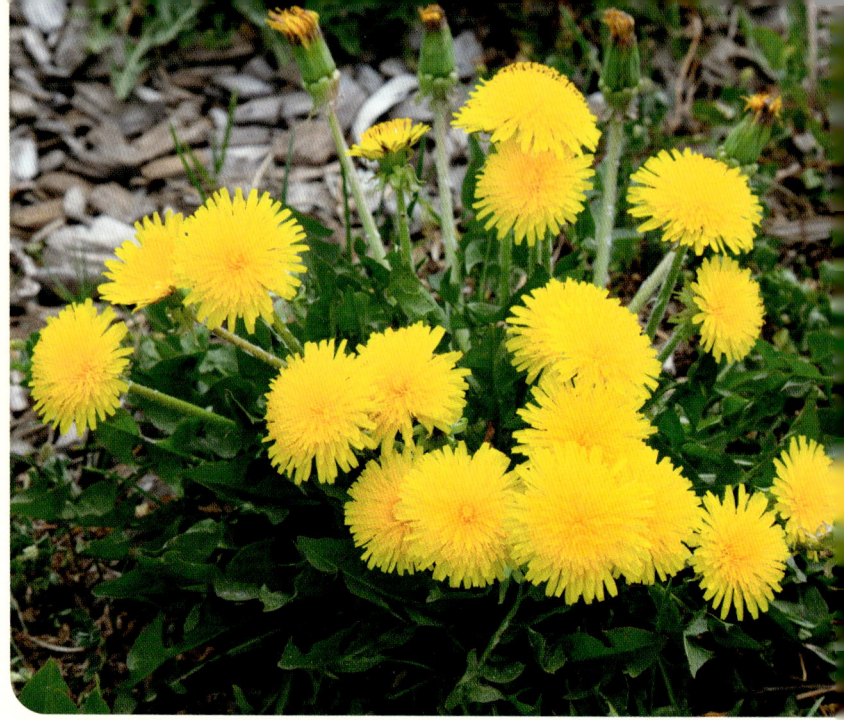

Foraging can be as simple as gathering a handful of dandelions from your yard.

I have been working with plant medicines for the past 10 years, learning from countless teachers and elders, and nature itself. I've started farming projects and educational programs and traveled the world continuing to learn from others on the same path. I'm excited to introduce you to the world of healing plants and share the lessons I've learned.

In the coming pages, you'll first learn how to forage responsibly, the basics of identifying plants, along with how and where to harvest them. Chapters 4 to 6 include profiles of some of the most commonly found and useful medicinal plants, with information on how to identify them, their medicinal uses, and how to process them. Toward the end of the book, you'll find step-by-step recipes for transforming foraged plants into powerful medicines and medicinal foods.

Many guides to foraging can seem complicated (so many Latin names), intimidating (do you have to be a triple Eagle Scout to even try this?), or even dire (eat the wrong thing and you're done for!). While there is much to learn, and it's important not to simply snack on random berries, foraging for medicinal plants is something anyone can do safely and effectively. And this book will teach you how.

ARE YOU SURE I WON'T DIE?

Despite the recent surge in popularity foraging has enjoyed, many of us have unconscious biases about the natural world and eating foods from the wild. Whether it's due to movies, literature, or a general wariness of the unknown, many people are hesitant and even scared of harvesting and eating wild plants. We have it ingrained in our minds that whatever is stocked on supermarket shelves is the best and safest food. And while there's much to say about the flaws in our food systems, I'll leave it at this: The act of foraging wild plants for food and medicine is ancient, regardless of how new we think it is or what sort of trend it may appear to be. When we make medicines with wild plants, we honor ourselves and nature in a way that nourishes the body, the spirit, and the land all at once.

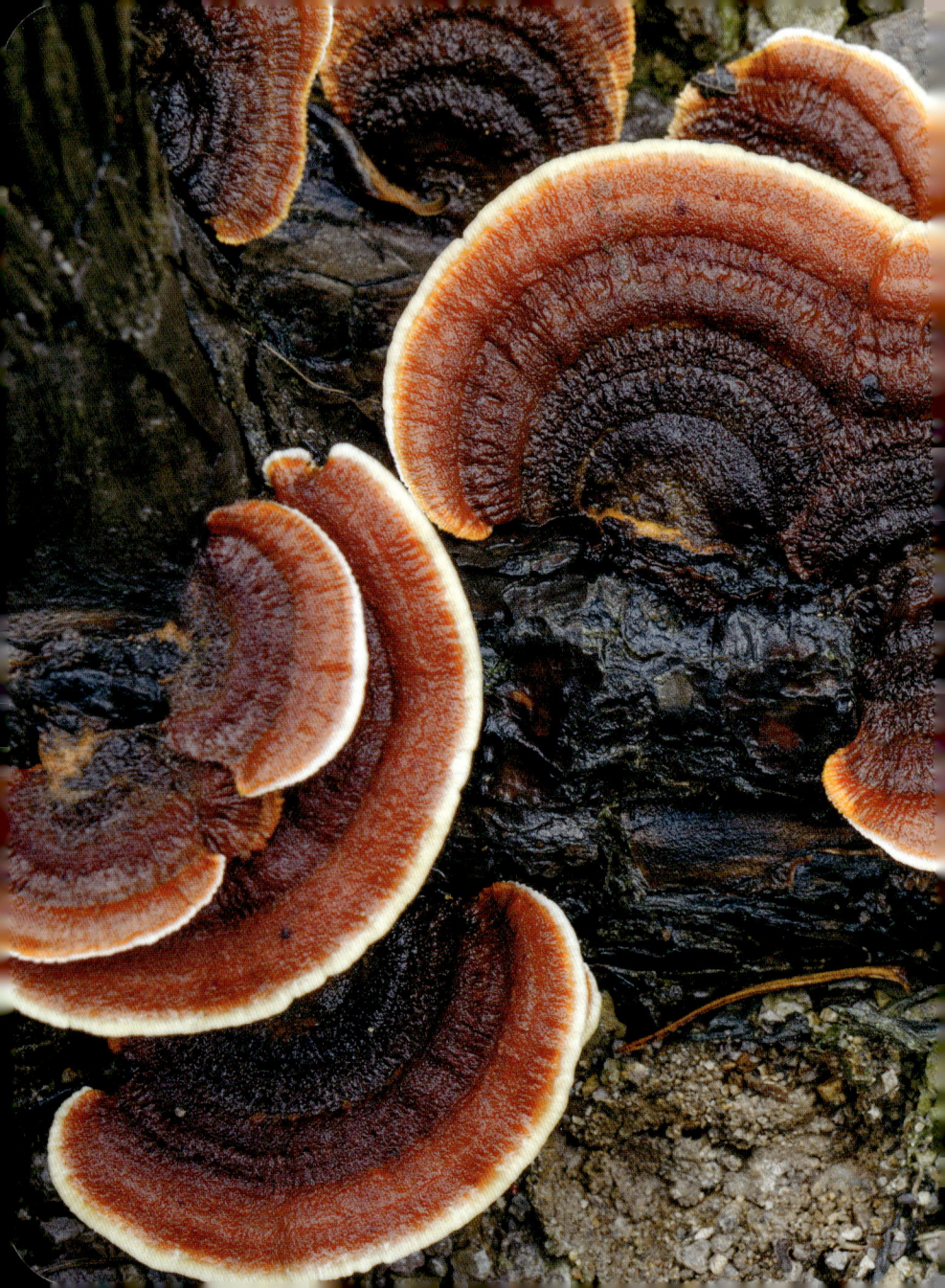

CHAPTER 1

RESPONSIBLE
Foraging

When we enter a wild place, we are stepping into an intricate ecological system that includes plants, animals, insects, and fungi, all of which have unique roles to play. To forage well, we must always understand what we are harvesting, why we harvest at different times, and how our actions affect the larger system.

Ethics in Foraging

Nature can seem vast and endlessly abundant. Yet the branches of trees, the root systems of shrubs, and some mosses may take years to grow just a few inches. When growth is slow, the impact of an uninformed forager can be dramatic and harmful; it is crucial that we approach foraging from a place of understanding and awareness.

When we forage we are extracting resources from the ecosystem. That's a sobering truth, but our goal is to forage in a way that is mindful and doesn't cause lasting negative disturbance. This means that in addition to harvesting responsibly, you shouldn't move large rocks or logs (especially in aquatic ecosystems), leave trash, or otherwise significantly alter a natural space.

THE IMPORTANCE OF ACTIVE STEWARDSHIP

Understanding is the key behind respectful and beneficial interactions with the natural world. While many of us love the idea of "unspoiled" nature, the notion that human intervention in the natural world is inherently bad is a consequence of colonialism and a failure to understand that humans are already a part of these intricate systems. For thousands of years in the Americas and all throughout the world, Indigenous people have been stewarding ecosystems and maintaining balance. For instance, the act of burning forests regulates and nourishes soil and plant life, and it was done for millennia. After colonization, fire was deemed inherently "bad," putting an end to this practice. Nature, colonists decided, was best left "wild." The consequences can still be seen today, with excessive wildfires raging across regions where controlled burns had once been used to add organic material and nutrients to the soil. With education, understanding, and initiatives led by those whose

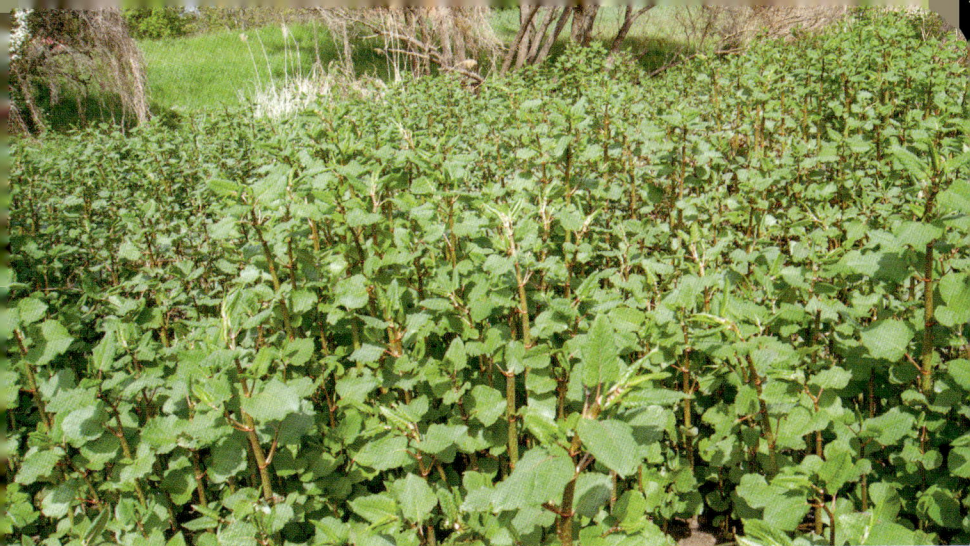

We can continue to steward the land around us by choosing to harvest invasive species like Japanese knotweed more heavily, helping to curb their growth.

ancestors have lived on these lands since time immemorial, we can steward our forests correctly.

As you begin your foraging journey, it's helpful to keep these two realities in mind: Yes, humans can, and do, harm the earth. But we are also capable of living in harmony with the natural world, tending to and caring for the ecosystems that support us and other living things.

SETTING INTENTIONS TO FORAGE RESPONSIBLY

What does it look like to harvest plants responsibly? The answer can depend on numerous factors, from the abundance of the species to the time of year and your purpose in harvesting. However, when you enter a natural environment, there are a few intentions and guidelines that are helpful.

RELEASE YOUR EXPECTATIONS. As you enter natural spaces, if you're hoping to gather a particular plant, try to release the expectation that you will find it. Setting your heart on finding one particular plant can lead to discouragement, or to harvesting plants you don't need to compensate for the disappointment of not finding "the one." The process of foraging is just as important as the product. A quiet walk in nature, observing plants in their natural habitats, is a healing experience, regardless of what you find. Don't hold so closely to your expectations that you lose sight of the beauty around you or trick yourself into harvesting what you don't need.

UNDERSTAND WHETHER A PLANT IS AT RISK. Before you forage, it's crucial to have some basic information about the plants you're looking for, especially whether a plant is endangered or at risk in a particular habitat. If a plant's wild populations are small and threatened by overharvesting or habitat loss, it should always be left undisturbed. It's our responsibility as foragers to research the status of the plants we hope to gather. The risk status of all the plants covered in this book will be mentioned so that you can forage wisely. See page 22 to learn more about native and nonnative plants and their role in the ecosystem.

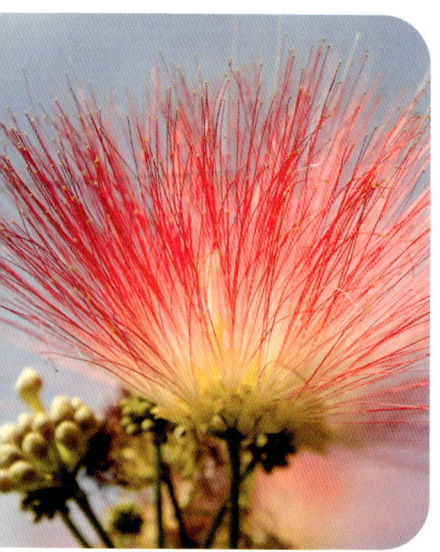

Though mimosa is often used in landscaping, it's actually invasive, making it an ideal plant to forage.

ONLY HARVEST WHAT YOU CAN USE. Always avoid wasting the plants that you harvest. At the beginning of my herbal journey, I harvested plants without considering this, eager to make medicine. Once I brought my harvest home, I'd find myself busy with work and other things, missing ingredients, or just distracted. Suddenly three days would pass and my leaves were moldy. When you forage, know how you will use the plants you harvest, so that you do not gather more than you need simply because you can. Do you have a space to dry what you forage? Do you have all of the ingredients needed to make medicine?

Once you've harvested a plant in the wild, a clock starts. If you want your plants to be fresh, delicious, and rich in medicinal constituents, make sure you're well equipped so that your medicine can go from bush to jar the same day.

CONSIDER THE PLANT. Before I harvest a plant, I often like to ask the plant for permission on both a spiritual and a practical level. Stick with me if you're skeptical about the "spirit" element. The spiritual act of asking permission also connects to the physical and practical. How does a plant "tell us" it doesn't want to be harvested? Pay attention to the environment and overall ecosystem. If you find the species of tree you've been looking for, but you realize it's the only one of its kind in the area, that is a clear indicator not to harvest from that tree. If you're harvesting leaves and see many specimens of a plant, you might take a handful of leaves from each plant. Avoid stripping a single plant of all its leaves, flowers, fruit, or seeds.

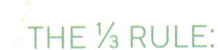

THE ⅓ RULE:

As a rule of thumb, only harvest from one in three of the plants you encounter.

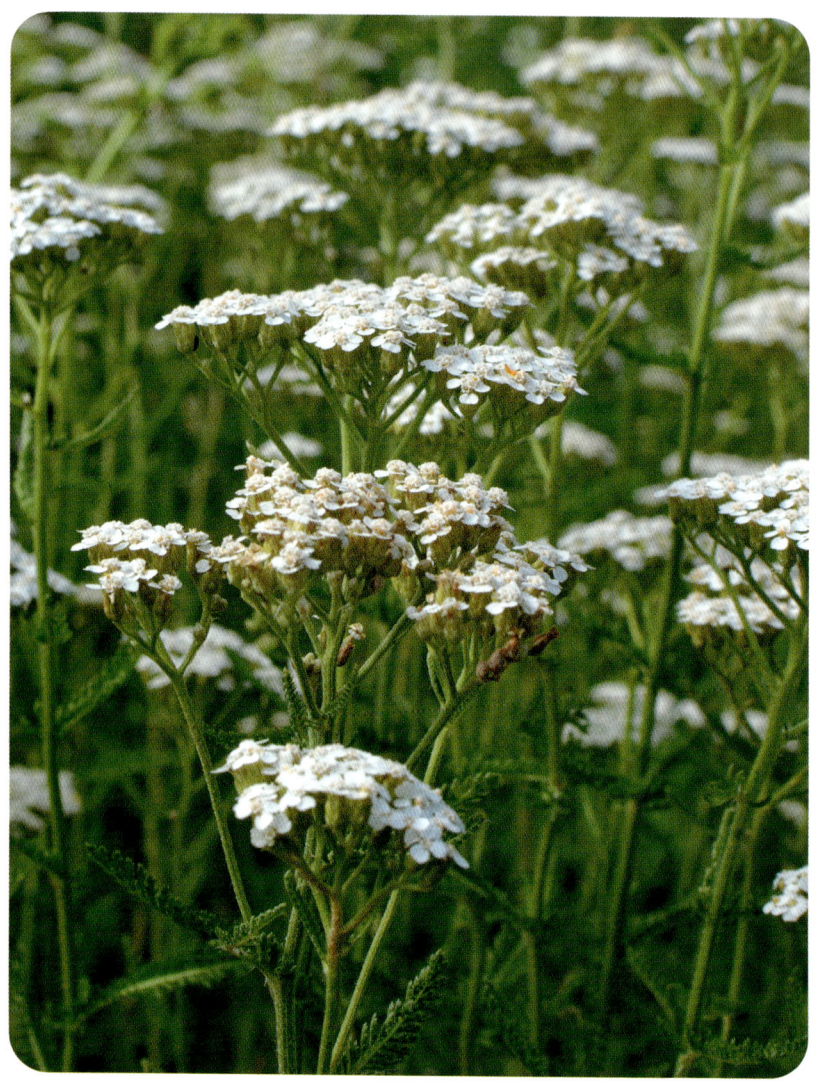

Remember, the plant needs to be able to survive and reproduce, the creatures must eat, and sometimes other humans may be looking for the same plants. Try using a rough ⅓ rule: If you find 10 plants, harvest from 3 to maintain the population.

STEWARD THE LAND. Foraging is a great opportunity to actively steward the environment around us. I love to care for the plants I encounter while foraging, especially if they're harder to find or even at risk. Years ago, while foraging for spicebush, I always took the time to spread the seeds of the blue cohosh and black cohosh growing nearby, knowing that they were rare in the area. You want to be able to return to your foraging spots for years, not carelessly exhaust them in a few seasons.

We are at a unique time in history when our wild spaces are threatened by environmental degradation, which makes it even more important that we have a reciprocal relationship with our environment. As you forage, ask yourself how you can support the ecosystem and plants you encounter. Spread seeds, pull invasive plants and vines that might be outcompeting native species, and seek to protect the plants that you find.

Responsible foraging requires that we understand the role a plant plays in an ecosystem. For instance, flowers like yarrow are an important source of food for pollinators of all kinds.

Native Versus Nonnative

A crucial part of ethical foraging is ensuring that you don't have a negative impact on the environment when you harvest a plant. For that, you need to understand a little bit about the role a plant plays in the environment. Let's go over some key terms.

NATIVE

A native plant is one that is naturally occurring in an area or region and is an integral part of the ecosystem. It plays a primary role in the health of the landscape and is interrelated with pollinators, insects, and other parts of the environment around it. Given their importance in the ecosystem, always harvest native plants mindfully, making sure that the population can continue to thrive.

ENDEMIC

An endemic plant is native to only a small, restricted region. Since their range is limited, these plants are more ecologically fragile. Avoid harvesting endemic plants, as they have a unique role in their ecosystem.

NATURALIZED

Naturalized plants have been introduced from elsewhere in the world and have adapted to their new environment over time, growing as if they were native and establishing themselves in large numbers. Dandelion (page 54) and plantain (page 66) are examples of naturalized plants that originated in Europe and now grow throughout North America. Many people see them as common weeds, but they arrived only a few hundred years ago. Ecosystems shift and change throughout history, and our human habit of taking plants along with us when we move results in the naturalization of plants. Most naturalized plants integrate into

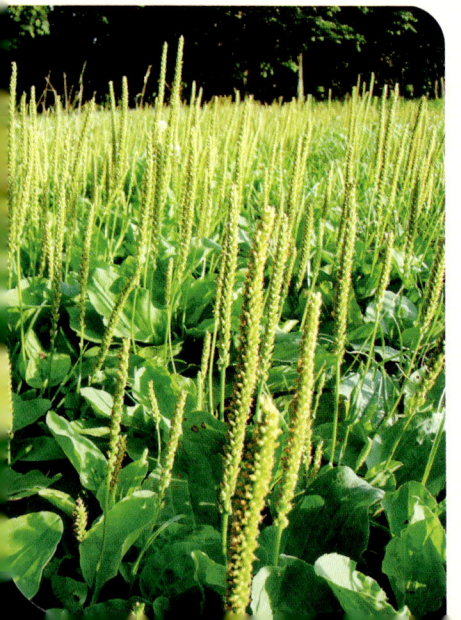

Plantain, also called white man's footprint, was brought to North America from Europe and has since become naturalized across the continent.

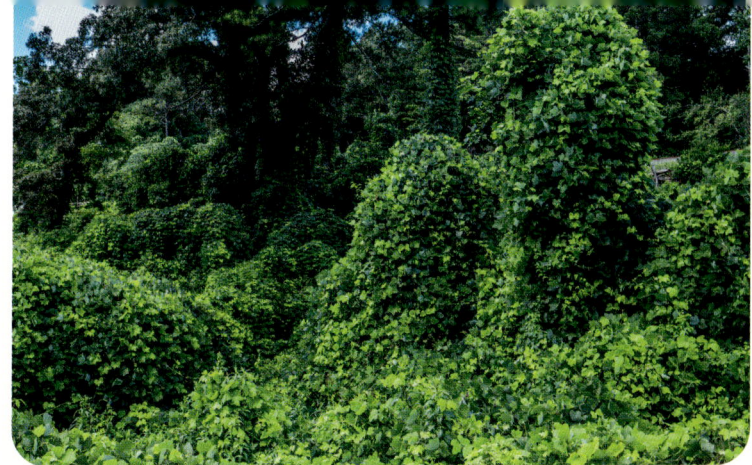

Kudzu is an example of an invasive plant with a detrimental impact on the landscape; it easily overtakes and smothers native plants and trees.

their new environment without posing a threat to the native ecosystem (more on that below), but I tend to harvest plants like these more often to allow more space for native plant growth.

INVASIVE

What a word! *Invasive* is a term used to describe plants that have been introduced from a different region and have a negative impact on their new ecosystems. Plants such as Japanese knotweed (page 83) and kudzu (page 87) come to mind, both of which are edible and medicinal among many other uses. The harm comes when invasive plants outcompete native species, threatening the ecosystem. While it's easy to blame the plants, remember that humans brought them to their new homes in the first place. The plants are just doing what they do best: growing.

Often these plants are "managed" by spraying toxic chemicals, which then damage the surrounding land and bodies of water. I believe that through educated environmental management and by harvesting invasive plants for their traditional uses, we can control and even eliminate some of these plants from our ecosystems. One of the easiest ways foragers can help control these plants is by harvesting them more heavily, allowing more space and nutrients for native plants to thrive.

In the following pages, you'll encounter a range of native, naturalized, and invasive plants. Knowing what these terms mean and understanding how these plants interact with the ecosystems around them will better prepare you to forage responsibly.

Ethics in Foraging

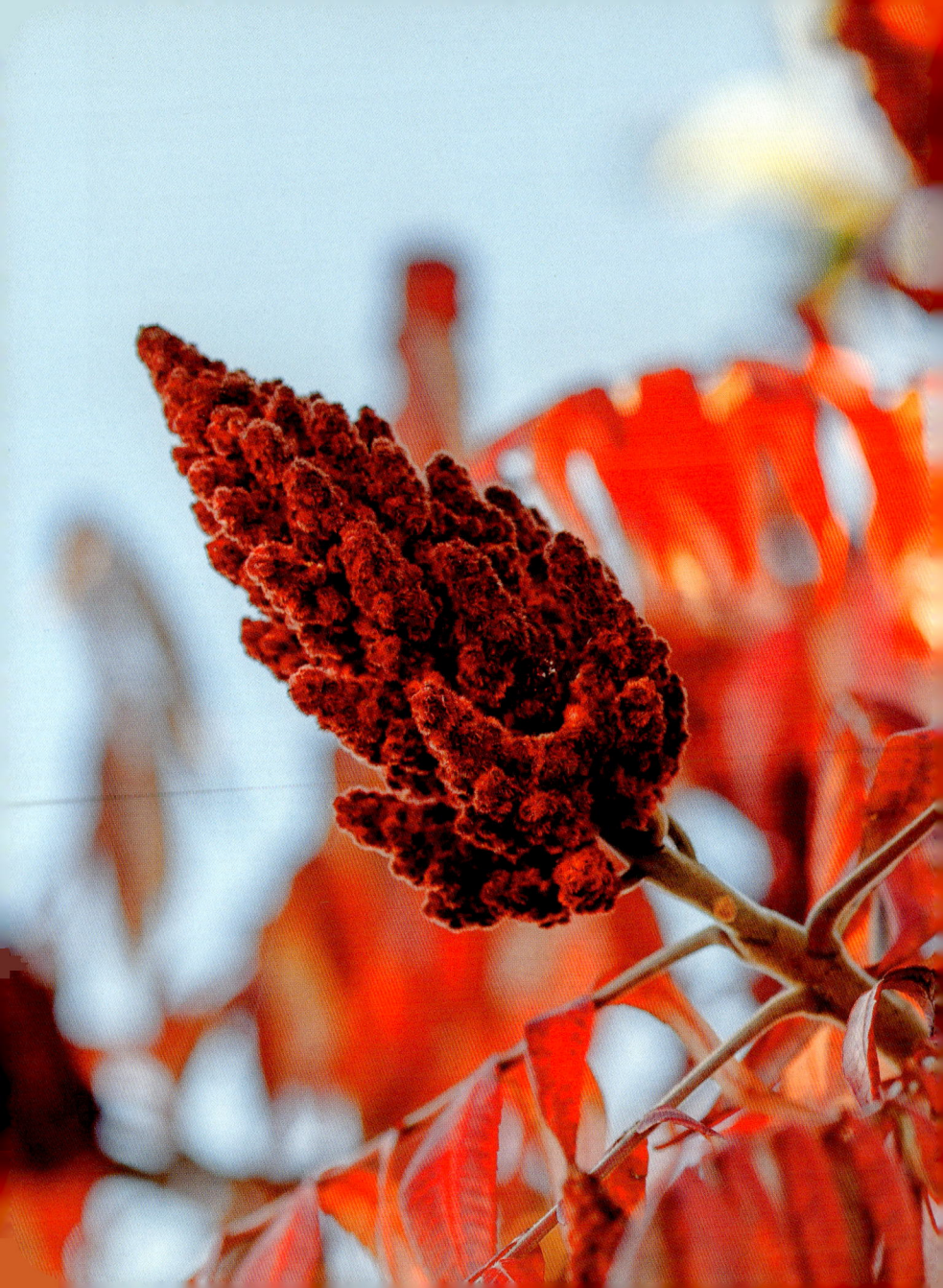

CHAPTER 2

How to IDENTIFY A PLANT

When you first begin foraging, the idea of learning to accurately and confidently identify a plant can be daunting. However, you'll soon discover that with a little bit of knowledge and observation, many of the plants around you will become familiar friends.

Combining Traditional and Technical Knowledge

Identifying plants is one of the most important parts of foraging. Throughout my years as an herbalist, I've used both traditional identification skills and technical botanical information to help me accurately ID a plant.

TRADITIONAL PLANT KNOWLEDGE is often experiential and can be invaluable as you begin to forage. The oldest herbalists on the land use visual and sensory cues to scrutinize and identify different plants. Listening to elders or community members, you may learn that a plant smells like mint, has spikes along the stem, or has yellow flowers in summertime. I've become familiar with many plants this way, learning out in the field alongside a knowledgeable teacher.

TECHNICAL BOTANICAL KNOWLEDGE can confirm and complement experiential learning by helping you understand plant families, specific descriptive terms, and contextual information such as a plant's range or conservation status.

By combining these two approaches you can confidently identify a plant. As you're learning about plants, be sure to talk to your elders and knowledgeable community members while also reading up on botany, so that you build both your practical "in the field" wisdom and your botanical knowledge.

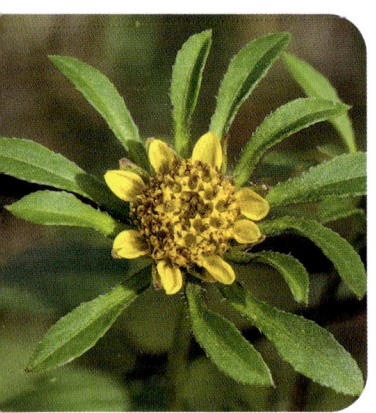

Learning about plants from community members is always valuable, particularly if a plant has a rich history of use in a community. Spanish needle, for instance, has been used in the Caribbean for generations.

The Importance of Proper Identification (i.e., Not Dying)

Positive identification is crucial in order to safely consume wild foods and medicines. Are you 98 percent or 99 percent sure you know what something is? Leave it. Unless you are completely, 100 percent certain that you have identified a plant correctly, you should not consume that plant. Some plants have look-alikes that might be toxic. You don't want to discover something is inedible as you're chewing it. The plants we'll learn about in this book are all common and relatively easy to identify, but that doesn't mean you can be careless or risky in how you forage.

ENVIRONMENTAL VARIABILITY

While some plants might be unmistakable, others have evolved together and they may look incredibly similar. Even with all the books and resources imaginable to help you identify a plant, the genetics, environment, and circumstances of an individual specimen can impact its appearance. Shapes, colors, and patterns can vary plant to plant. All of these things together conspire to make identification tricky.

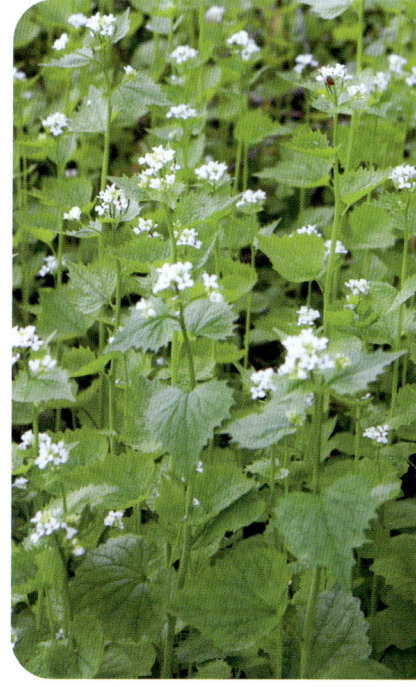

Biennials like garlic mustard look very different in their second year of growth, making it even more important that you are familiar with their habits before you harvest.

Knowing your particular bioregion will help you understand what you can expect to find in your area. However, sometimes a plant will pop up in your region that you've never encountered or that generally grows somewhere totally different. It's just a matter of a bird eating a seed thousands of miles away and happening to poop it out near you (hopefully not on you, though!).

This book is a beginning primer on some of the most common and useful medicinal plants, but there's a world of abundant resources you can make use of. Reach out to your foraging community, read other books, and look at online resources to be sure of your identification. If you're not sure about a plant, use three confirmations: a plant identification book, a trustworthy person knowledgeable on the subject, and online resources.

Using Plant Identification Apps

While plant identification apps are helpful and can be efficient, they are not always 100 percent correct. I've seen an app identify the new growth of poison hemlock as "wild parsley"—not a mistake you want to make! Apps might be one tool in your identification arsenal, but don't rely on them alone to make a positive identification.

Plant Anatomy

Now that you're probably too scared to identify so much as a blade of grass, let's talk plant anatomy. Keep in mind that all plants are different, and their anatomy can be wildly complex; this is a basic primer and not a PhD text in botany. But these basics will get you well on your way to identifying and foraging confidently.

ROOTS, RHIZOMES, BULBS, AND TUBERS

Most people will dig up a plant and call the brown things roots, but in reality there are different types of underground structures.

ROOTS. Plants can have either sprawling root networks or taproots, single roots that grow deep into the ground and hold most of the nutrients in a plant (a carrot, for example). Regardless of what form they take, roots attach the plant to the ground, offering support and drawing in nutrition and water. Many, like garlic mustard, are medicinal.

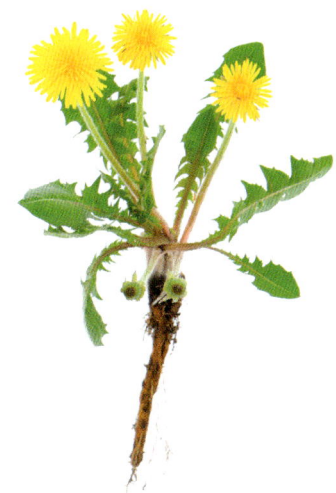

RHIZOMES. These play a key role for many plants by storing energy. They may have some small rootlets growing off of them, but they're really an underground stem growing horizontally that can sprout and create a new plant entirely. Ginger (*Zingiber officinale*) and Japanese knotweed (page 83) are good examples. Rhizomes tend to be significantly larger than other roots.

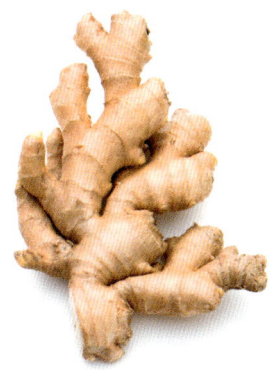

BULBS. Plants like onions and wild garlic produce bulbs. These plants grow one spherical underground stem with small roots at the base. They may reproduce with new bulbs or by seeds aboveground.

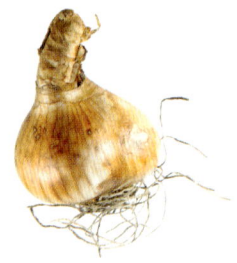

TUBERS. Plants like potatoes or dahlias grow tubers, usually sprouting directly from the roots. Tubers serve as an underground energy storage system for the plant. Kudzu (page 87) has tuberous roots that are notoriously hard to eradicate.

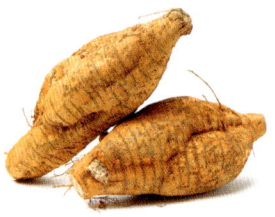

STEMS

Stems are the main structures of a plant that support leaves, flowers, and fruits. Many plants have leaflets growing off of the stem, but sometimes the leaves grow directly on the stem, such as cleavers (page 58). Older stems, those lower on the plant, tend to be tougher and fibrous. The more fibrous the stem is, the fewer medicinal compounds it tends to have, so it's generally better to cut higher up, close to the new growth. New shoots are often good medicine, such as stinging nettle (page 151), which is vibrant and fresh in spring when it first emerges.

Harvesting stems usually involves cutting most of the plant, so be mindful if you want the plant to produce fruits and seeds later in the year. Harvesting midseason can help stimulate more growth later in the year, encouraging the plant to branch out and get bushier.

LEAVES

Leaves are the parts of the plant that enable it to photosynthesize, drawing energy from the sun's light. They are often the harvestable part of the plant and are used in many medicines. Leaves can vary in thickness but tend to be easy to process and dry for medicinal purposes. The freshest, newest leaves are ideal for medicine making, as they often have the highest concentration of medicinal constituents. Many leaves are also aromatic, with a distinctive smell, which can be helpful when identifying a plant.

FLOWERS

These lovely structures emerge from a plant in various colors and shapes to attract pollinators. Some bloom at night, others throughout the day, depending on the pollinator needed. Both flower buds, which are closed and yet to unfurl, and open blooms are used for medicinal purposes, depending on the plant.

Flowers tend to be the most tender and least shelf-stable part of a plant, drying out easily or degrading with too much heat or time before being used. Flowers are usually aromatic, and these aromas are best captured in oils, teas, steams, or honeys. Preparations that require excessive heat, such as decoctions, can inadvertently destroy this aromatic quality. Each flower is different, but the thinner the petals and more fragile the bloom, the more easily its medicinal qualities are lost when it's not processed correctly.

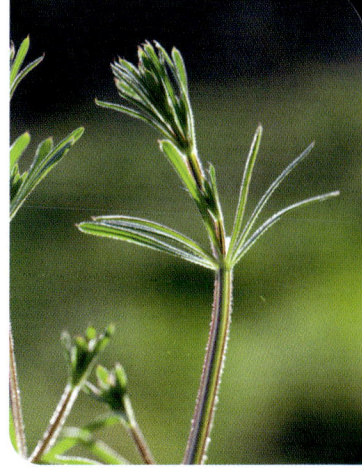

The leaves of cleavers grow directly from the stem, which provides the central support for the plant.

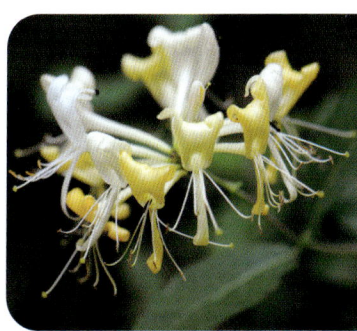

Many flowers, like Japanese honeysuckle, are delicate and should be processed as soon as possible to capture their aromatic qualities.

Leaf Identification 101

Leaves are more than just the green things on a plant. They're essential for photosynthesis and one of the primary ways that you can accurately identify a plant. These are some of the key terms used to describe and identify leaves.

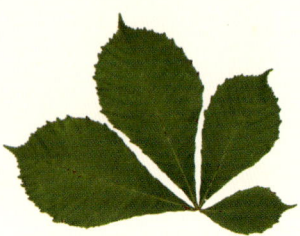

PALMATE. A palmate leaf has lobes originating from a single point and resembles the palm of a hand.

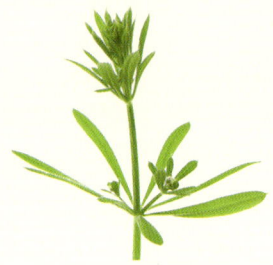

WHORLED. Leaves that grow in a circular arrangement around the stem of a plant are whorled.

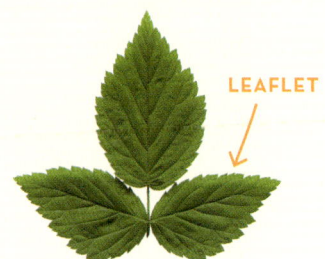

COMPOUND. These leaves are composed of smaller leaflets, which grow on their own stalks and emerge from a central stem. A **LEAFLET** is an individual segment or part of a compound leaf. Different species can have anywhere from 2 to 24.

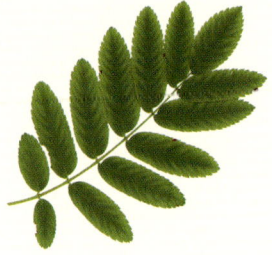

PINNATE. The word *pinnate* comes from the Latin *pinnatus*, meaning "feathered." Pinnate leaves do indeed resemble feathers, with leaflets on both sides of a central stem. In *bipinnate* leaves, the leaflets themselves are also compound.

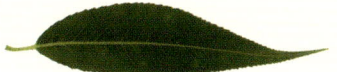

LANCEOLATE. Longer than they are wide and usually tapered to a point at the end, lanceolate leaves resemble the head of a lance.

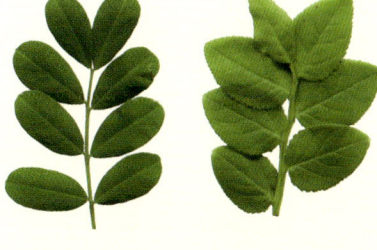

OPPOSITE. These are leaves that emerge as pairs on opposite sides of the stem (pictured above left).

ALTERNATE. These are leaves that grow one by one in a staggered pattern, alternating sides along the length of the stem (pictured above right).

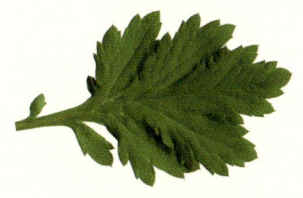

LOBED. Leaves that have lobes or divisions extending at least halfway to the center are lobed.

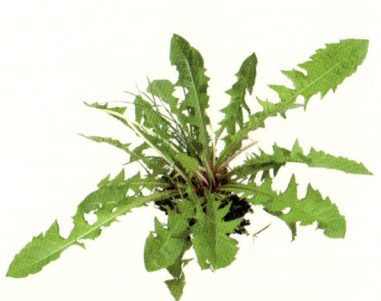

BASAL. Leaves emerging from the same point in the ground, sometimes pointing upward or laid out flat on the soil, are basal.

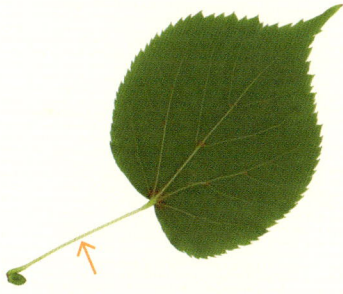

PETIOLE. This is the stalk that attaches a leaf to a stem.

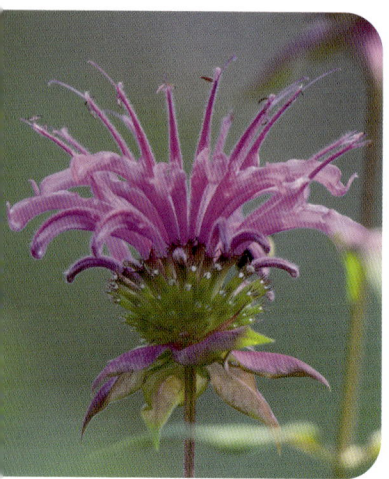

The calyces of bee balm are rich in aromatic compounds.

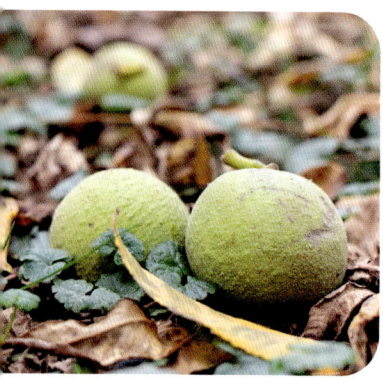

While the nuts of the black walnut tree are delicious, the husk surrounding the nut is the part that is used medicinally.

CALYCES

Calyces (*calyx*, if there's just one) form a protective layer over the budding flower, sometimes remaining on the plant until fruit has formed. For example, the stylish green hat on an eggplant is a calyx. Many calyces contain potent medicine; bee balm (page 160), for instance, is medicinal when using just the petals, but the green calyx is also rich in aromatic compounds key to the plant's healing properties.

FRUITS

From an evolutionary standpoint, fruit is the culmination of a plant's life cycle. Dropping ripe fruit filled with seeds ready to germinate is the final step of reproduction for many plants. As a fruit ripens it will often soften, change color, or simply fall off the plant. Make sure you're aware of the properties and edibility or inedibility of the seeds; the fruit may be edible but not the seeds. The various components of the fruit (rind, skin, juice, seeds, etc.) can often be used in different ways and require different processing. For example, when using black walnut (page 146), the hull of the fruit is medicinal, while the nut inside is a delicious edible treat.

SEEDS

Seeds usually develop at the end of the plant's life cycle as a means of reproduction. Seeds can be dried relatively easily and some, like plantain, dry right on the plant. If you're working with a native plant, especially one that isn't abundant in the wild, be sure to leave a few plants for other creatures to use, and to ensure the production of new plants next year.

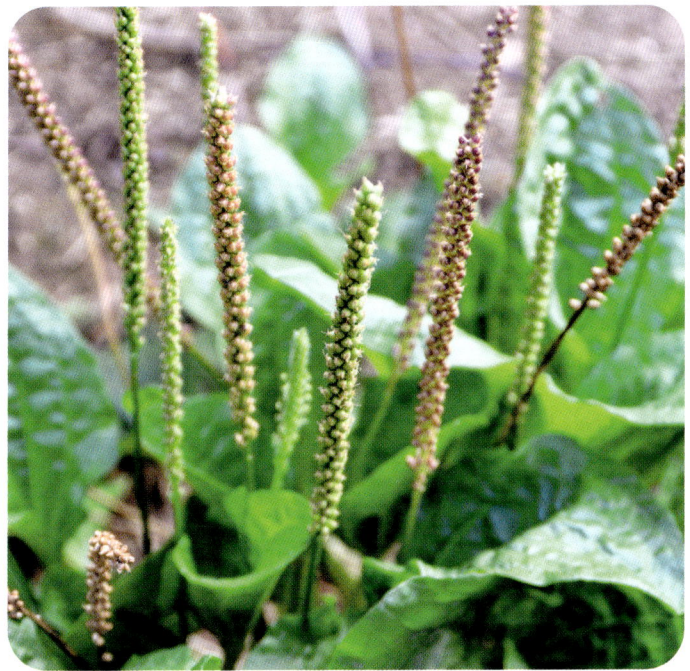

Dried plantain seeds are a great source of fiber.

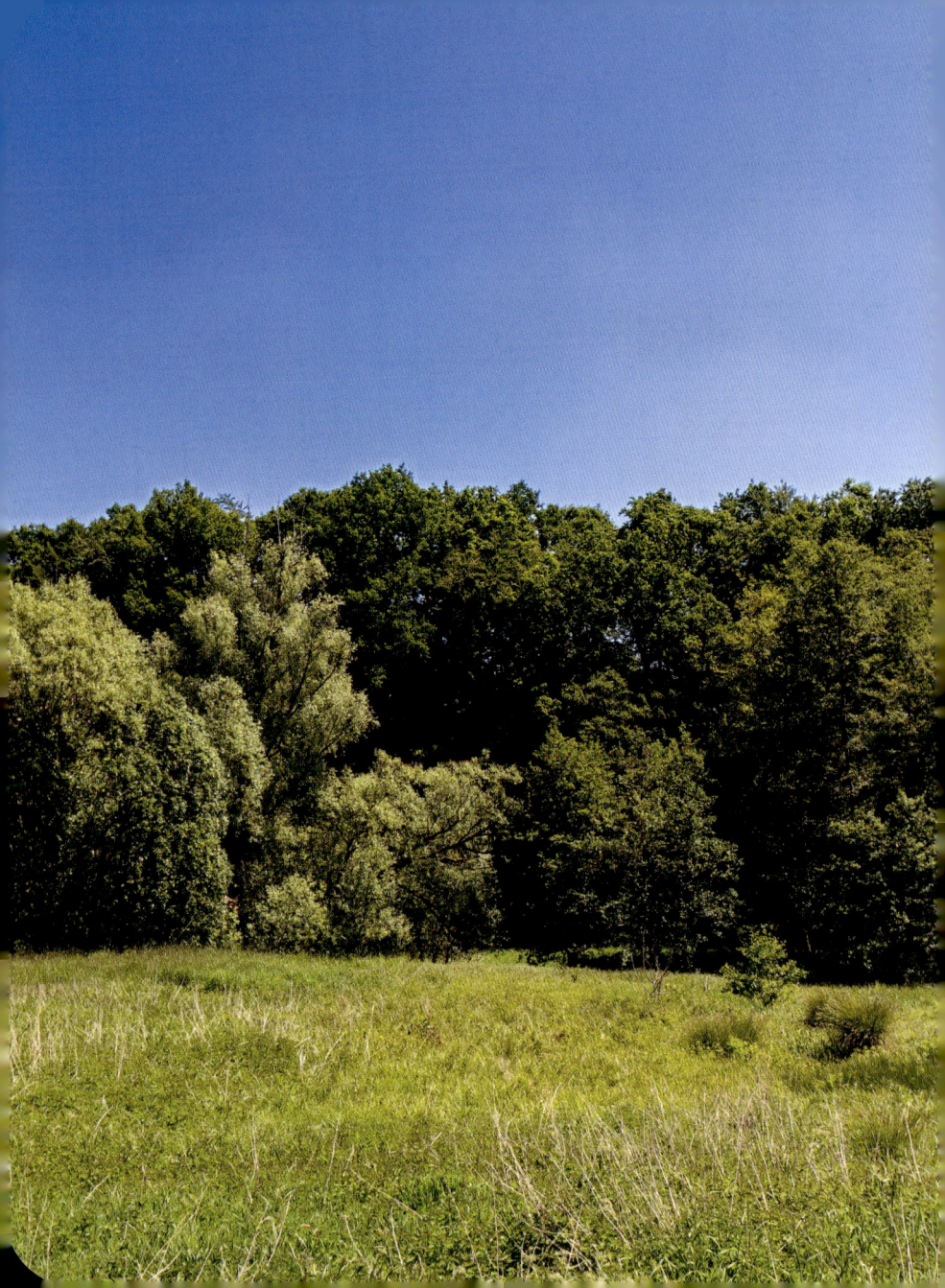

CHAPTER 3

What to Bring, WHERE TO GO, AND WHEN TO FORAGE

Now that you're armed with a basic knowledge of plant identification terms, we can focus on getting out in the field. But which field? Or forest or neighborhood park? And what do you need to bring along with you? Let's explore some essential foraging tools and learn where to forage.

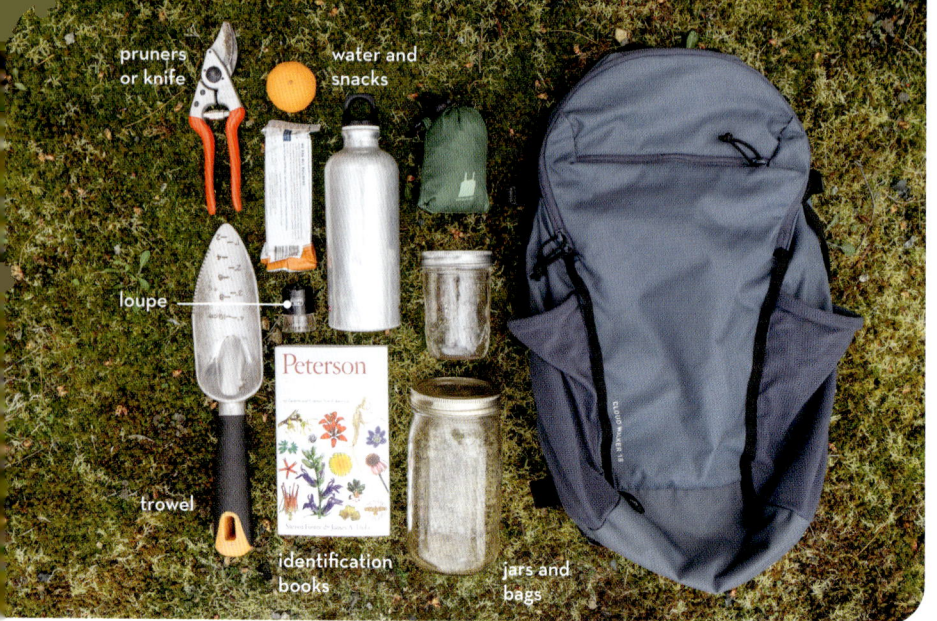

Tools for Foraging

Before you head into the woods to harvest medicine, you'll want to be properly equipped. This means having the right tools, understanding where you can forage, making a plan for what you want to gather, and having the knowledge to harvest responsibly. These are some of the tools I use most frequently and that you'll want to have on hand as you venture out.

PRUNERS OR KNIFE

When harvesting a plant, the goal is to make clean cuts and to avoid twisting and damaging the plant. A clean cut makes it easier for the plant to direct energy away from that node, stimulating future growth. I prefer handheld pruners from a hardware store, as they cut stems and small branches easily. If you prefer a knife, the Opinel brand is excellent. However, knives are better suited for leaves and easy-to-cut stems rather than woody stalks or branches.

Occasionally I bring a machete with me, but there are some pros and cons to doing this. Pros: Nobody will bother you. You can cut anything from tree bark to leaflets, and on the off chance you're wandering into an area known for sword fights, you'll be prepared. Cons: Walking around with a machete is sure to raise eyebrows and perhaps alarm a park ranger. So I generally just stick to pruners and a pocketknife. Whatever you choose, make sure to keep the cutting edge sharp and handle it with care.

JARS, BAGS, AND BASKETS

You'll need something to easily and safely carry your harvest. I've tried throwing dirty roots, fungi, and branches directly into my backpack, and I would not recommend it. Jars or baskets are ideal for fragile things that will otherwise be crushed in transport, such as berries or flowers. Bags work well for barks, branches, and leaves. Plastic bags are usable, but I prefer cloth to help prevent mold growth and decomposition. A sturdy, spacious backpack, with lots of pockets and compartments, is ideal for carrying all your tools, containers, and eventually your harvest.

IDENTIFICATION BOOKS

Along with this book, which is of course coming with you on all your foraging outings, it's never a bad idea to have an additional identification book, whether it's a technical book specific to your region or another popular book by an herbalist and forager. Having multiple visual references can be helpful to ensure that you identify a plant correctly. The Peterson field guides are excellent and are available for many different regions.

LOUPE

A loupe is essentially a small magnifying glass, and it can come in handy for looking more closely at the details of a plant. A loupe can easily be put on a string and worn around your neck for convenience. I like to use mine to look at tiny insects, fungi, and flowers to see the small features that might not be visible with the naked eye. Some identification books list features that you won't be able to see easily without magnification, so a loupe is a great tool. You can buy one at your local outdoor store or online.

TROWEL

A trowel is helpful for harvesting roots and tubers. A hori hori is ideal for foraging. It's a Japanese agricultural tool that's similar to a trowel, but one side has a blade to allow for cutting. Since harvesting from the ground is often particularly destructive to a plant, always be mindful: Consider seasonal cycles and ethical harvesting.

WATER AND SNACKS

Don't forget to stay hydrated and have something in your stomach! Always carry more water than you think you might need—foraging can be thirsty work.

Staying Safe

When foraging, all the basic rules of outdoor safety apply. Know where you are and your route home, go with a friend or at least inform someone of where you will be and when you expect to return, dress for the weather, and avoid being caught out in the dark. Leave no trace. And never do anything Smokey Bear wouldn't approve of!

Where to Forage

Medicinal herbs are growing all around us! Many of our plant allies are powerfully resilient and able to adapt to a variety of climates and growing conditions. Still, it's important to carefully consider where you're foraging before you begin. We want to make sure our medicines are sources of natural healing that are free of toxins or harmful chemicals.

When I first began foraging and working with wild plants, I would forage just about anywhere. You could find me off the side of the highway with a friend, shouting over the noise of cars rushing by about how great goldenrod (*Solidago* spp.) is for sinuses, or in a parking lot delaying our night out in the city by showing everyone how resilient wild lettuce (page 110) is as it grows through the concrete. But in subsequent years, I've become much more thoughtful and considerate about where I forage.

RESIDENTIAL AREAS

Parks or residential areas are common spots for foraging. While these locations are easily accessible, plants and landscapes in these places are subject to the whim of their owners and can be sprayed with pesticides, rat poison, fertilizers, and other chemicals you don't

Where Does It Grow?

The majority of plants featured in this book grow abundantly across North America and often in other places around the world as well. The specific range of each plant is included in the plant profiles in Chapters 4 to 6.

want to get into your medicines. Before you forage in residential areas, it's important to learn about potential pesticide or herbicide use. For all you know, those lovely looking dandelions you were hoping to harvest were just sprayed with weed killer. And while rain can wash off surface pesticides and herbicides, the roots of the plants can still absorb many different compounds. Some plants are even dubbed *hyperaccumulators*, meaning they are capable of absorbing heavy metals and other pollutants from the soil and holding onto them. Not something you want to be making tea with!

If you spot an abundant harvest in a yard or on private property, always ask the homeowners before foraging, both for permission and to ensure that no chemicals have been sprayed on the plants. When speaking with a property owner, offering to bring them some of the harvested plants or some of the finished medicine in thanks can be a great way to build community.

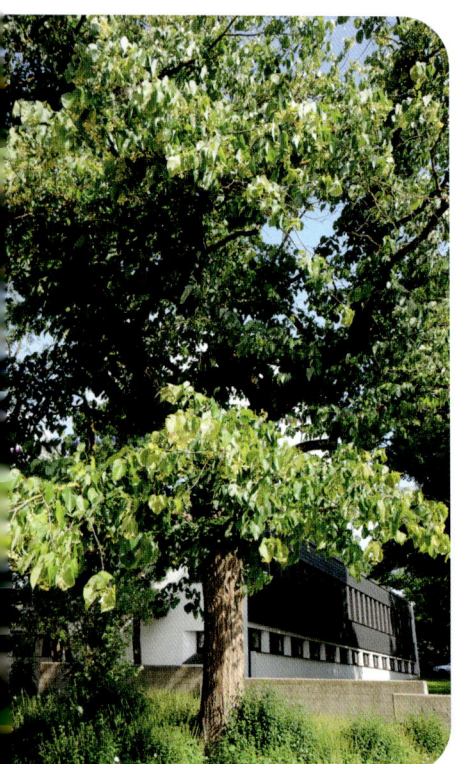

Some species, like linden (page 190), are commonly planted in residential areas and cities.

FORESTED LAND

In residential neighborhoods, it's often easy to identify property boundaries and know which door you need to knock on to ask permission. Undeveloped land can be trickier. You still want to be sure you aren't trespassing on private property or other areas where someone has the legal right to ask you to leave. When approaching forested land, look for areas away from residences to ensure that you're not bothering anyone in the neighborhood. In the end, communication is key. Asking is always better than sneaking around hoping to avoid being detected. I've developed many friendships and connections by simply asking people if I could forage in the area.

PARKS AND PRESERVES

Foraging in national and state parks and nature reserves can seem like an obvious choice, but according to many laws and regulations it's illegal to remove plants, objects, and other natural features from these places. These restrictions are intended to protect natural resources, endangered species, and delicate environments, which is particularly important when you consider that many national parks have millions of visitors each year. However, some parks do allow foraging in particular areas or in small amounts, so it's always worth inquiring.

AVOID HIGH-TRAFFIC AREAS AND ROADWAYS

As tempting as it may be, it's best not to harvest plants in high-traffic areas. The soil along roadsides may have accumulated chemicals from the asphalt or via runoff from vehicles on the road, which can be absorbed by the plants growing there. Also, these areas are commonly sprayed by the county or state for "weed prevention." Spraying is especially common in areas with invasive plants such as kudzu (page 87), where the vines can destroy telephone towers and other structures along the road. You can sometimes tell if an area along the forest or roadside has been sprayed if the first few feet of plant life is dead or discolored. Oftentimes, officials won't spray deep into the forest but just on the very fringe. However, the pesticides can still run off into nearby ditches and drainage, affecting the ecosystem and other plants nearby. So be mindful!

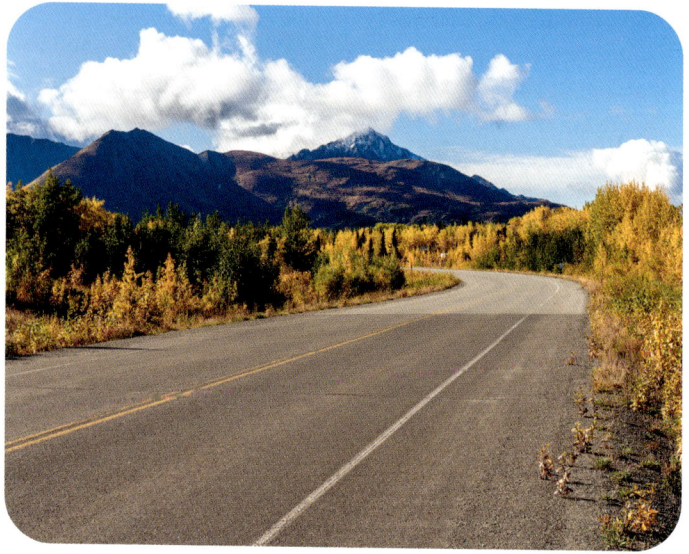

While roadsides can seem like ideal places to forage, the plants growing there are often exposed to chemicals from the asphalt or passing vehicles.

Foraging in Transitional Zones

Roadsides are what ecologists call "transitional zones"—areas where one type of landscape or terrain changes to another. Even though it's not a desirable place to forage, many medicinal and edible plants thrive in the transitional space between forest and road. Fortunately, you can look for the same type of ecological transition elsewhere, such as where forests meet meadows or ponds.

This "edge" is a unique place where sun exposure, water availability, and the overall environment change, encouraging new plants to grow. At a spot near my home, honeysuckle vines cover red raspberry bushes, transitioning into burdock and garlic mustard at the edge of the forest. These transitional zones are a unique aspect of the ecosystem that we can train our eyes to see.

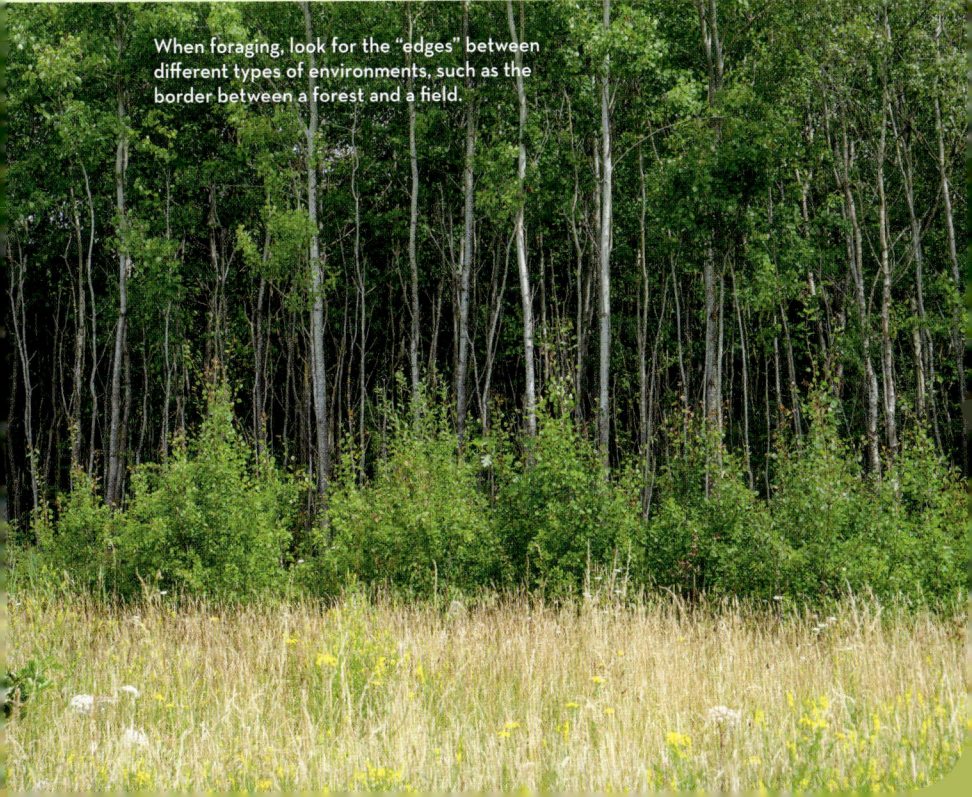

When foraging, look for the "edges" between different types of environments, such as the border between a forest and a field.

When to Forage

In the course of a year, a plant will use its energy differently. In spring a plant sends its first shoots out, growing gradually and putting energy into foliage and stem development. When summer arrives the plant has already established its root system, leafed out, and devoted its energy to the aerial parts of the plant. Over the summer months, the plant begins to bloom, channeling energy into developing flowers to attract pollinators. Once the flowers have been pollinated, the plant begins developing fruit. When ripe, the fruits contain mature seeds that will reproduce the plant. The plant may continue to produce additional flowers and fruit throughout the season. As the weather cools, the plant begins to move its energy back into the leaves and stem and finally to the roots as winter comes.

The cycle can vary depending on the plant and the climate, but this general process is a good blueprint to keep in mind as you consider the ideal time to harvest.

CHOOSING WHEN TO HARVEST

When you forage will depend greatly on the plant species and your own region and climate, in addition to the part of the plant you're seeking to harvest. However, these general guidelines can help you time your harvest to ensure you're gathering a plant at its peak.

ROOTS. These are often best harvested in fall or early winter, when the plant is gathering its energy underground before the coming season of cold and dormancy.

STEMS. Look for fresh growth when harvesting stems, as they can become fibrous and woody over time. Spring and summer are generally the ideal times to gather stems, but be mindful that a plant may

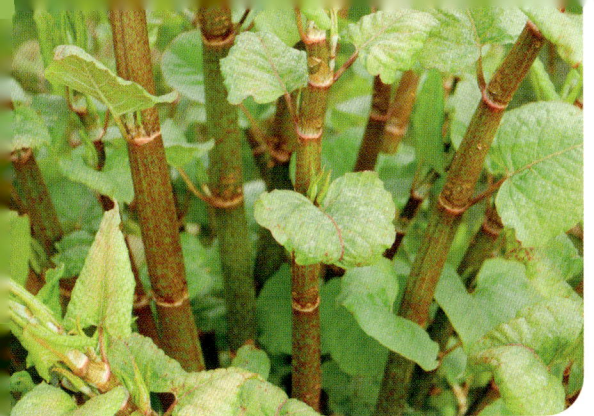

Japanese knotweed stems are best harvested when they are tender young shoots, before they become too tough to enjoy.

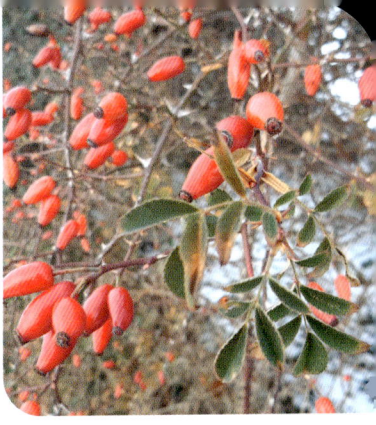

Rose hips can linger on the plant long into winter, allowing them to be harvested for many months.

not produce flowers, fruit, or seeds depending on how extensively you harvest the stems.

LEAVES. These are present throughout most of the growing season or all year, depending on the plant and region. New leaves generally have the highest concentration of medicinal compounds, so spring and summer are often the best times to gather them. Avoid harvesting older, dried leaves or right before the plant loses its leaves in fall.

FLOWERS. The timing of the harvest will depend entirely on when the plant blooms, but for most plants that will be spring or summer. Harvest flowers within a day or two of opening, when they are at their most aromatic.

CALYCES. The timing of this harvest will also depend on when the plant blooms and fruits. Calyces can be harvested young, before fruit or seeds have developed, or separated from the fruit later in the season.

FRUITS. Generally, plants will produce fruit at the end of the growing season—late summer through fall. The ideal harvesttime will depend on the plant. Some fruits, such as black walnut (page 146), are best harvested before they're fully ripe, while others, such as rose hips (page 133), offer more flexibility. Fruit can rot quickly or be devoured by birds and other hungry critters, so keep an eye on its development throughout the season.

SEEDS. These are the final step of the plant's reproductive cycle. Seeds are often harvested once they've dried on the plant itself, as with plantain (page 66). You can plan to forage them toward the end of the growing season, sometimes even into winter. If you're harvesting seeds inside a fruit, they will be at their most potent when the fruit is completely ripe.

Cleaning and Preserving

If you don't want a creepy crawly floating in the middle of your mug of reishi tea, you'll need to clean your harvest. Apart from removing rogue bugs, thoroughly cleaning foraged plants ensures that dirt, gravel, and other substances don't end up in your finished medicines.

If you have access to an outdoor source of clean running water, washing your plants outside can avoid a mess in your kitchen.

While washing plants is necessary, it also introduces excess water, which can make them more susceptible to molding and spoiling. After cleaning, plan to use the plant immediately or make sure that it's thoroughly dried.

LEAVES AND FLOWERS. Place a bowl in your sink and fill it with water, submerging the plant material and gently agitating it. Refill the bowl as needed, washing particularly dirty leaves under a stream of water. If there are deep grooves in the leaflet or petiole, you can use a toothbrush to remove any dirt. Be careful not to rip or crush the leaves while washing them. Flowers are particularly fragile, so handle them with care and avoid holding them directly under the faucet.

ROOTS AND STEMS. A toothbrush or nail brush (designated just for cleaning plants) is a great help here, allowing you to get into the nooks and crannies. Roots and stems are generally sturdy, so you can use the spray feature on your faucet to clean them. The crown of the root where the shoots emerge is often curved and full of crevices that can benefit from a good brushing and spraying.

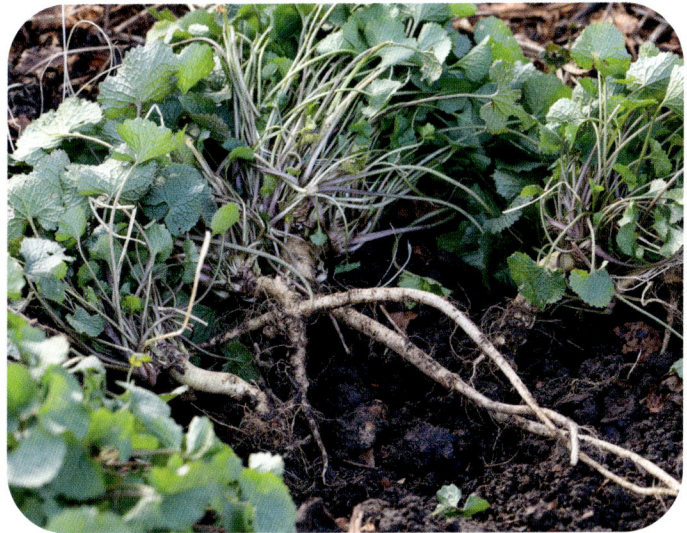

Many roots will require a good scrubbing with a toothbrush or nail brush.

NUTS, SEEDS, MUSHROOMS, AND BARKS. These plant parts are more durable and can withstand a good scrub and soak. If you're concerned about insects or worms in your harvest, allow the plant material to soak for a few hours to eliminate any stowaway bugs. Be sure to dry your plant material well or use it immediately, as it will have absorbed water while soaking.

PRESERVING YOUR HARVEST

While using fresh plants is great, sometimes you'll want to preserve your harvest for the future. Many plants are harvested in spring and summer (see page 46) but can be used for ailments in other times of the year, easing a winter cold or offering immune support during flu season. Finding a way to preserve your seasonal harvest can allow you to enjoy plant medicine year-round.

DRYING. Drying herbs is one of the best ways to preserve them for future use. A dehydrator is a helpful tool for drying foraged food, as it can be set to a specific temperature depending on the plant material and will provide reliable results. Roots, barks, and fruits dry best in a dehydrator. Particularly moist fruits, such as those of mallow (page 141), can benefit from being cut into pieces before being dehydrated. If you don't have a dehydrator, try preheating your oven at its lowest temperature setting, then turn it off and place plants inside to dry in the residual heat, or use your oven's "proof" setting.

More delicate plant material such as leaves, stems, and flowers can also be air-dried. If you're air-drying a plant, harvest it with a length of stem still attached and hang it in a well-ventilated area out of prolonged direct sunlight. Check on it every few days to ensure

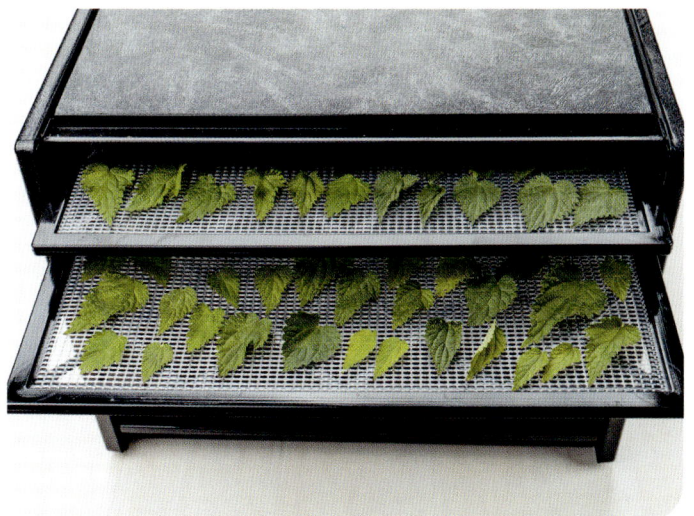

A dehydrator is an excellent way to preserve spring plants, like stinging nettle, for winter usage.

it hasn't begun to mold or mildew. Most plants will dry in a week or so; you'll know they are completely dry when you can easily break off a piece or crush it in your hand.

FREEZING. Freezing works well for fruit or berries, but I wouldn't suggest it for leaves or other plant materials, which can be damaged by the freezing and defrosting process. You can also freeze your finished medicinal preparations if they are water based.

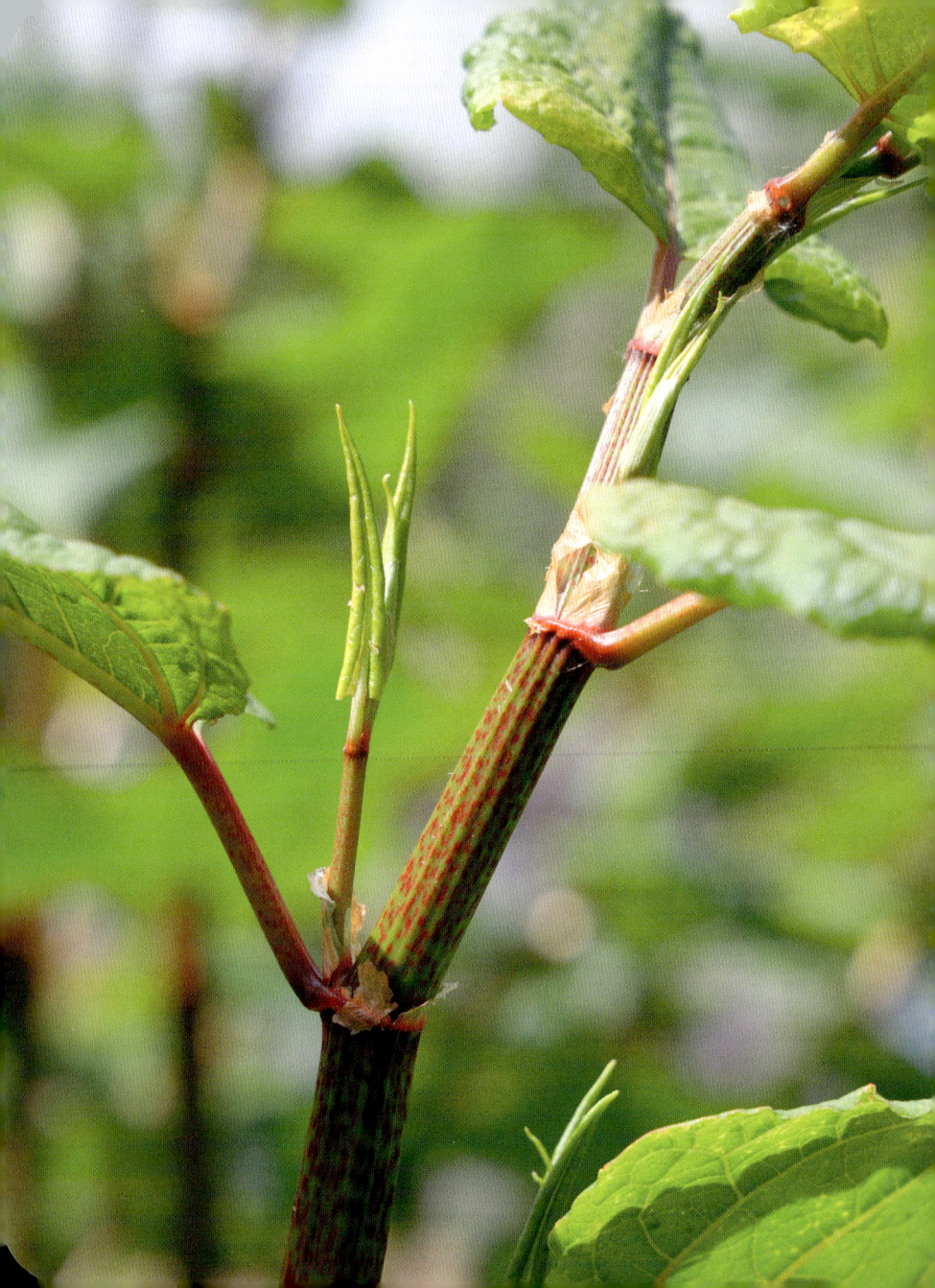

CHAPTER 4

Wonderful WEED MEDICINE

It turns out that some of the most common and frequently maligned plants are also sources of incredibly powerful medicine. As you begin to forage and make plant medicine, you'll soon come to see these "weeds" in a new way.

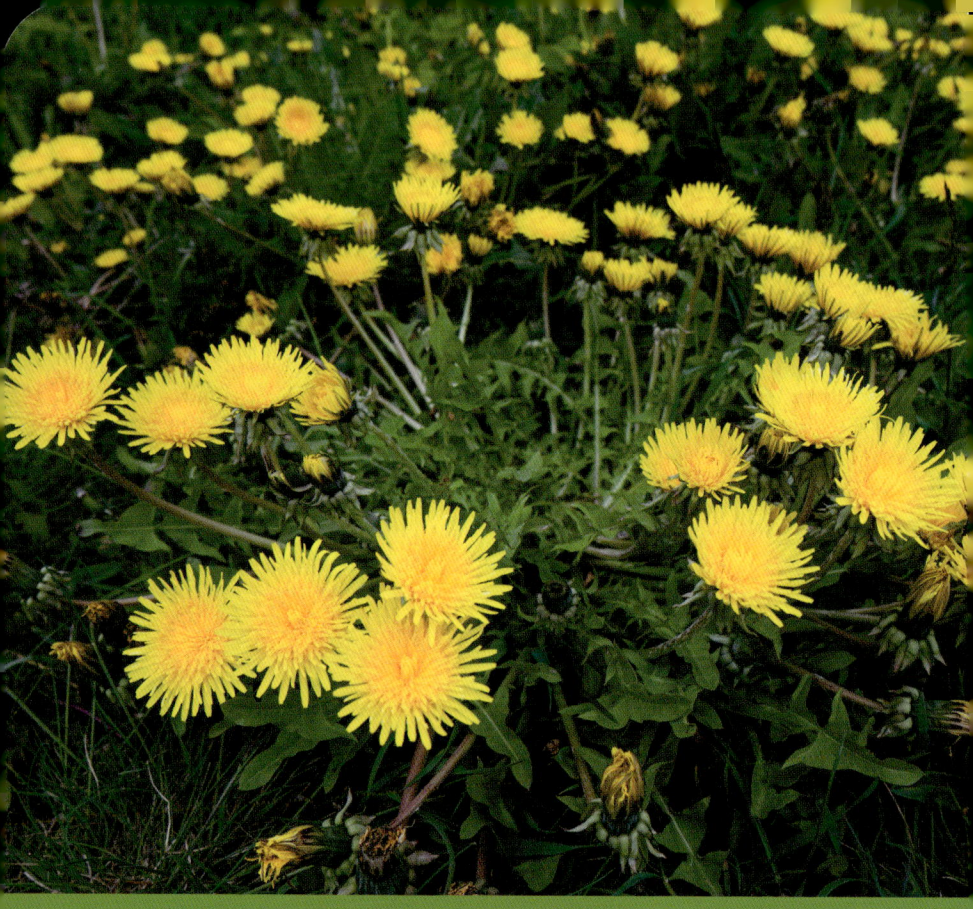

DANDELION

Taraxacum officinale
Family: Asteraceae

Other Names: blowball, dent de leon, pissabed

Parts Used: leaves, roots, and flowers

When to Harvest: spring and fall

An icon of the herbal world, dandelion represents resiliency, strength, and the power of nature. Often seen growing through cracks in the concrete and in industrialized areas, this plant ally grows all around us. Originally from Europe, it's naturalized in the Americas and used in herbal healing traditions around the world. From the flowers to the roots, the entire plant can be eaten and made into medicine. Dandelion is a bitter remedy that helps us regulate our systems, especially when we tend to gravitate toward sweet and salty instead of bitter flavors.

BENEFITS

Bitter. Stimulates digestion and acts on the liver

Diuretic. Helps the body eliminate excess water through increased urination

Choleretic. Helps increase bile production and encourages elimination of toxins

Nutritive. Rich in vitamins and minerals

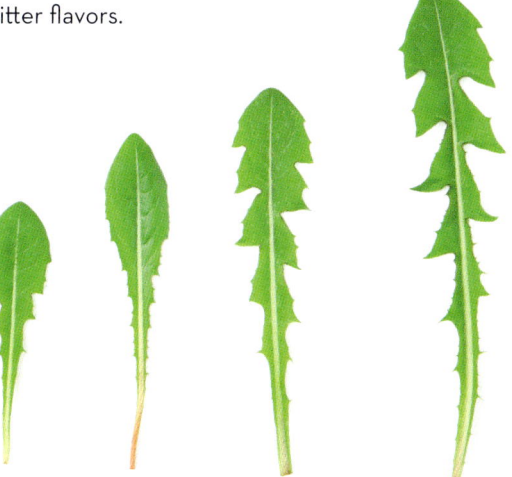

The shape of individual dandelion leaves on the same plant can vary.

IDENTIFICATION

Dandelion grows from a basal rosette, sprouting leaves from one central point, and commonly grows with its leaves close to or on the ground. Unlike some of its look-alikes, such as cat's ear (*Hypochaeris radicata*), dandelion's leaves are hairless and mildly to deeply lobed. Individual leaves on the same plant can look very distinct. The serrated edges of the leaves point outward or back toward the base of the plant. Dandelion develops a large taproot and a single, bright yellow flower.

Cutting the hollow stem, leaves, or flowering stalk will release a white latex, a distinct characteristic of dandelion and an important aspect of its medicinal quality. This latex is bitter and helps nourish the gut. After blooming, the flower will dry into a globe of dried seeds that spread by wind or if you blow on them to make a wish. Dandelion is a short-lived perennial that reseeds each year and can tolerate many different climates and environmental conditions.

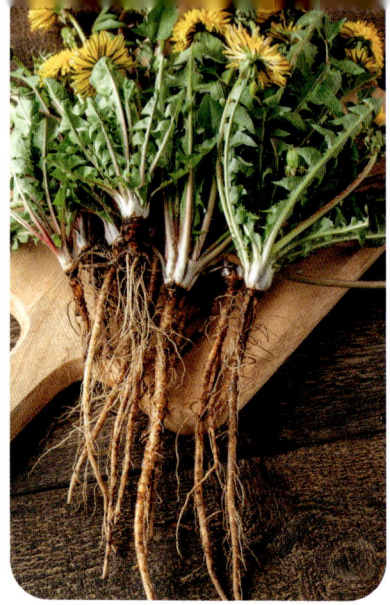

Dandelions have a long, edible taproot.

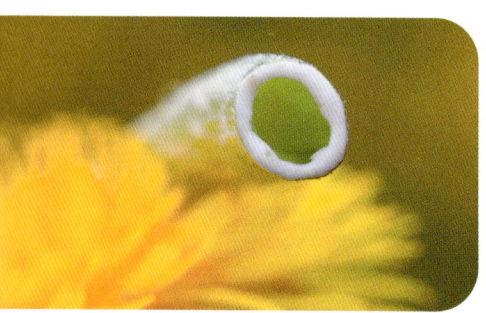

When cut, the stem, leaves, and flowering stalk of a dandelion will ooze white latex.

TRADITIONAL USAGE

Dandelion traditionally has been used as a bitter tonic for the digestive system. The entire plant, from flower to roots, is used, and its bitter flavor helps stimulate digestion, ease discomfort after eating a heavy meal, and regulate digestive flow. Dandelion emerges in early spring and is the perfect medicine to help you recover from winter, moving stagnant blood and reviving energy in the body after a long season of cold.

The leaves can be eaten as a potherb and salad green or boiled to make tea. The roots are used in tinctures, boiled, or eaten as a powerful diuretic that also nourishes the liver. Rich in the prebiotic fiber inulin, the raw and cooked roots of dandelion also support probiotic bacteria and can help maintain gut health. The flowers can be boiled fresh or dried to make a bitter tea. In some parts of the southern United States, they are battered and fried as a tasty treat.

HARVESTING

It's best to harvest dandelion leaves before the plant flowers. Cut the leaves directly from the center of the plant. The root is best harvested once the flower has dried out and the plant has focused its energy back to the root. The plant will flower multiple times throughout the season; gather the flowers when they are fully blooming and open but before there are any signs of drying on the petals. Make sure you know your harvest area is clean and free of herbicides, as dandelion will grow anywhere and is often treated as a weed.

PREPARATION

As a nutritious green, use dandelion like any other leafy green, washing and chopping as needed and adding it into various recipes. You can try incorporating the leaves into pesto, green goddess dressing, or other flavorful sauces if you dislike the flavor but want the plant's nutritive benefits. The leaves make an excellent tea; drink it throughout the day to take in the nutrients and that wonderful bitter medicine. The flowers can be tossed into salads and eaten raw. Though dandelion root is edible raw and cooked, I prefer to tincture the root to concentrate its liver- and gut-nourishing properties. The tincture can be taken any time of year, but it's particularly beneficial in spring and fall.

DANDELION FAST FACTS

- Leaves are basal, growing along the ground or erect
- No leaves on flower stem, just flower
- Leaves are hairless with serrated edges pointing outward or back toward center of plant
- Harvested spring through fall
- All parts of plant used and can be eaten raw or cooked
- Can grow in polluted areas; harvest in areas that haven't been impacted by runoff from roads or pesticides

CLEAVERS

Galium aparine
Family: Rubiaceae

Other Names: stickywilly, catchweed

Parts Used: stem and leaves

When to Harvest: early spring

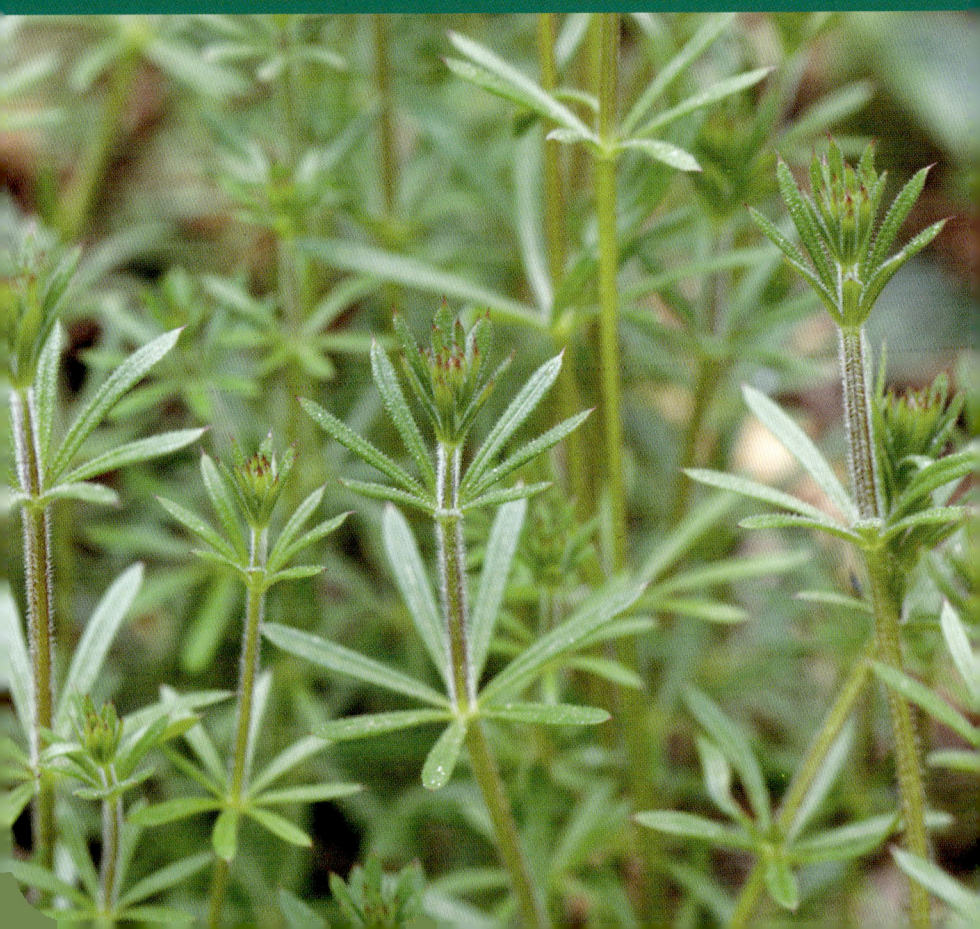

Take a walk through the forest and you might find cleavers has hitched a ride, sticking to your shoes and clothing like the botanical version of Velcro. Cleavers is a common plant, popping up in spring in grassy areas, yards, and many garden beds. Native to Europe, Asia, and northern Africa, this plant has long been used for medicine. Like many other herbs emerging in spring, cleavers helps us adapt to the season, cleansing the system and rejuvenating the body after a cold winter.

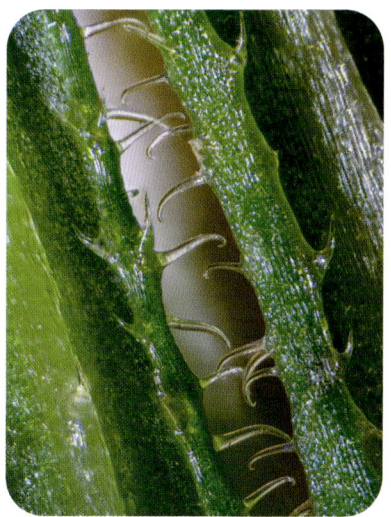

Cleavers is covered with fine, Velcro-like hairs.

BENEFITS

Lymphatic. Stimulates lymphatic drainage

Astringent. Tonifies skin and smooth muscle tissue

Diuretic. Helps the body eliminate excess water through increased urination

IDENTIFICATION

Cleavers is an annual plant that self-seeds. It grows abundantly in fields or disturbed areas across North America, first appearing in early spring and dying off by early summer. It has whorled leaves that grow around the stem along the length of the plant in groups of six to eight. The square stems and leaves have a distinct stickiness sometimes compared to Velcro. This is due to small, angled hairs that cover the plant's surface. You'll often notice cleavers sticking to your clothing or skin.

The flowers are white with four petals, indicative of the Rubiaceae (coffee) family. The seeds ripen to a brown color and are also covered in sticky hairs. Since cleavers is a member

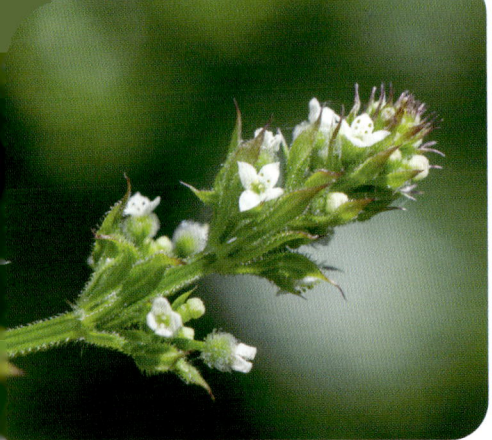

Cleavers has small, white flowers with four petals.

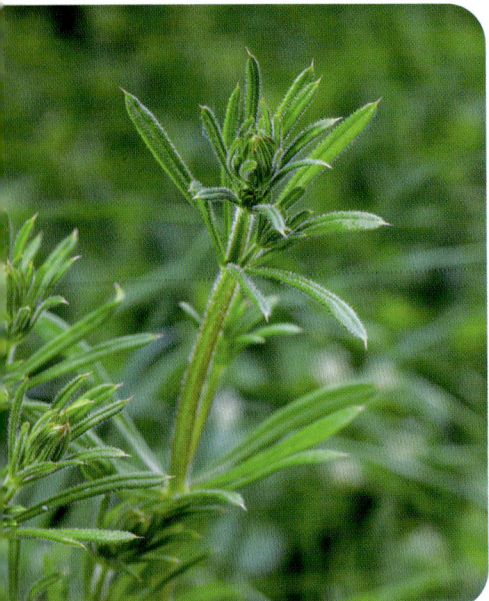

The leaves are whorled and grow directly from the stem.

of the coffee family, the dried seeds actually contain a small amount of caffeine! The plant usually grows sideways or as a mat, rarely growing upward unless supported by other plants or objects nearby.

TRADITIONAL USAGE

Cleavers is a cooling, soothing medicine that is gently stimulating and helps regulate our bodies in times of transition. It can be used as a refreshing spring cleanse, as it emerges in early spring and tends to die a few months later. Cleavers is a powerful lymphatic tonic, stimulating lymphatic drainage and moving the waters of the body as a diuretic and alterative. This is especially important in early spring, when our bodies may be moving a bit slower as we emerge from winter and colder temperatures. Our lymph nodes can swell when our bodies are fighting off illness; cleavers can help the body properly drain and cleanse these nodes. Cleavers is traditionally pressed for its juice, which is drunk regularly during spring. It can also be used as a soothing demulcent that helps cool hot ailments of the urinary tract such as UTIs and urethritis.

HARVESTING

Cleavers tends to grow abundantly in large patches and is best harvested in early spring once the plant grows about a foot tall. Harvest it while the plant's energy is focused on the leaves and stems, before the flowers dry and seeds start to form. I cut at the base of the plant, letting the stickiness hold the bundle together in my basket or backpack.

If you're making a tincture, a few handfuls of the plant will do. If you'll be juicing it, more is better. Try to gather at least half a pound of fresh plant material, or the equivalent of a large grocery bag fully packed. You'll still probably end up with much less juice than you anticipated.

PROCESSING

Cleavers can be harvested and dried; this is usually how the plant is sold commercially. However, I find the dried leaves to be less effective than the tincture or juice. To tincture fresh cleavers, you won't need to add water, as there is plenty in the stems. Just be sure to crush it or roughly chop it to increase the extractable surface area.

To make juice, simply wash your plant well (see page 48), then add it into the juicer. If you don't have a juicer, place well-chopped cleavers into a blender with a small amount of water to extract the medicine. You can keep this juice in the refrigerator for up to a week and a half. I sometimes make so much juice that I'll freeze it into ice cubes, drinking it whenever I want a cooling herbal beverage.

CLEAVERS FAST FACTS

- Entire plant is covered in fine hairs that latch onto clothing and skin
- Leaves are whorled around central stem
- Stem is square
- Best harvested in spring
- Common in disturbed areas, on the edge of forests and in garden beds
- Leaves and stems are used medicinally and can be eaten without cooking if tender

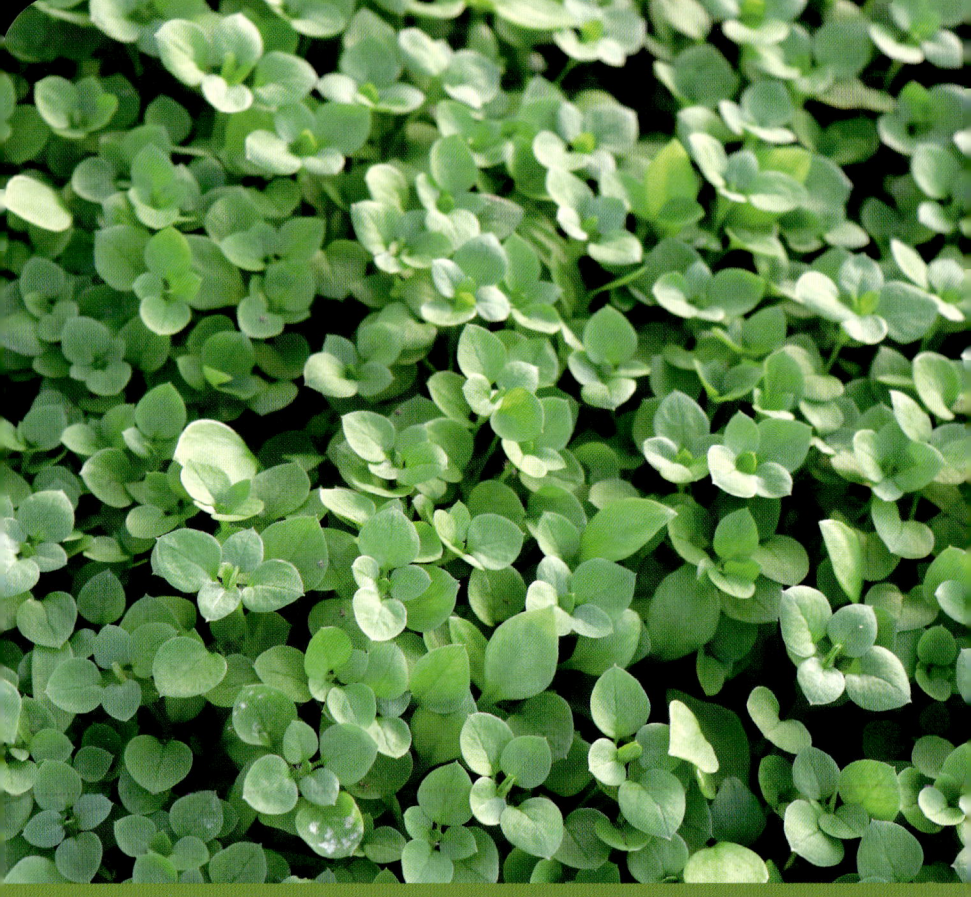

CHICKWEED

Stellaria media
Family: Caryophyllaceae

Other Names: birdweed

Parts Used: stems and leaves

When to Harvest: throughout the year, but preferably spring

I was first introduced to chickweed when it appeared as an unexpected visitor in the garden. An unknown herb kept popping up and sprawling through my garden beds alongside my holy basil and beans. I discovered it was chickweed, and instead of pulling it, I added it to my diet! Eating it, infusing it, and even making tea—the possibilities were endless. Originally native to parts of Europe and Asia, chickweed can be found across most of North America and has become a staple in my medicine cabinet and kitchen.

BENEFITS

Demulcent. Cooling and soothing

Nutritive. Rich in vitamins and minerals

IDENTIFICATION

Chickweed grows low to the ground and sprawls out across the ground, usually radiating from one central point. If it's supported by nearby plants or objects, the leaves can also grow erect, reaching 6 to 12 inches. This plant has a line of fine hairs growing along the square stem that alternate sides after each leaf or node. The small white flowers emerge at the top of new

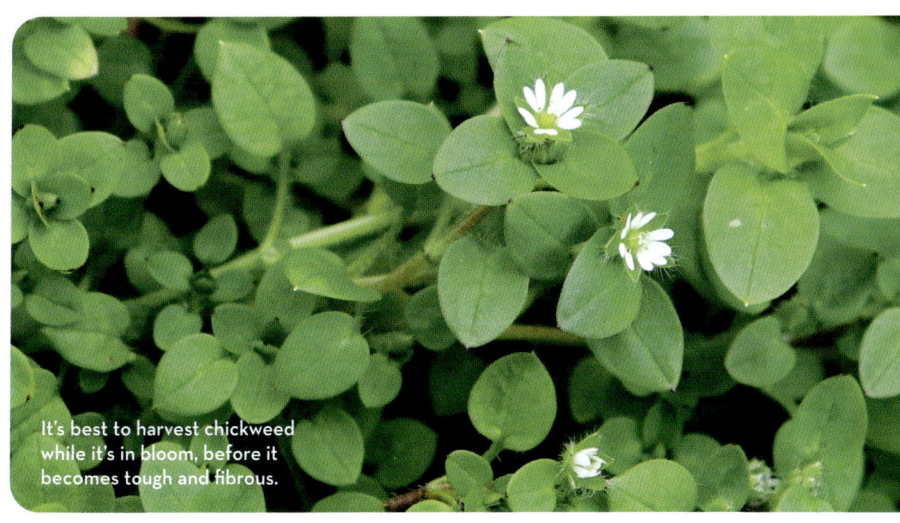

It's best to harvest chickweed while it's in bloom, before it becomes tough and fibrous.

Chickweed

growth and have about 10 petals each. The leaves are small and rounded in shape, with pointed tips. They grow on opposite sides of the stem in an alternating pattern.

TRADITIONAL USAGE

Chickweed can be used both fresh and dried but is best used fresh for skin ailments and as food. As a salad ingredient, the new growth has a mild herbal flavor that takes on whatever other flavors it's combined with. As a cooling demulcent, chickweed can be used internally and externally for hot conditions such as respiratory infections, upset stomach, rashes and bug bites, and even eczema. Chickweed is high in water content and easily exudes juice when squeezed, making it ideal for topical applications. Fresh leaves can be crushed and applied as a poultice to inflamed skin or dried and infused into an oil for topical use.

Chickweed is rich in minerals such as calcium, potassium, and copper, along with vitamins C, A, and B. This makes it a great addition to your seasonal diet;

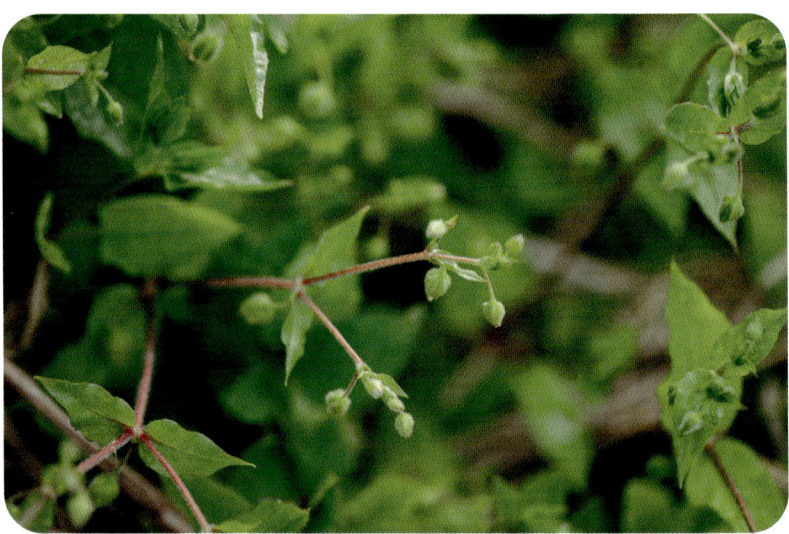

Chickweed is a great topical medicine and can even be made into juice, as it contains a lot of moisture.

incorporate it into your meals throughout spring, whether cooked or raw. As an herbal remedy, it combines well with other herbs to provide nutrition and a cooling energetic.

HARVESTING

If you have an abundance of chickweed, you can simply pull the entire plant up to harvest it. It's best to harvest chickweed while it's flowering, as it becomes a bit fibrous afterward. However, it is still usable at that stage. If you want to stimulate more growth, harvest it at the base of its basal growth, cutting the stems off so that it comes back soon after.

PROCESSING

Chickweed tends to be a bit juicy, so either dry it in a dehydrator or hang it in a warm spot with good airflow. Once dry it can be used for tinctures or making an herbal oil. If you want to use it for a poultice or as a fresh ingredient, use it immediately after harvesting. Fresh chickweed can be tinctured in alcohol. The dried plant can be used this way as well; simply add a bit of water to rehydrate the plant material (see page 214).

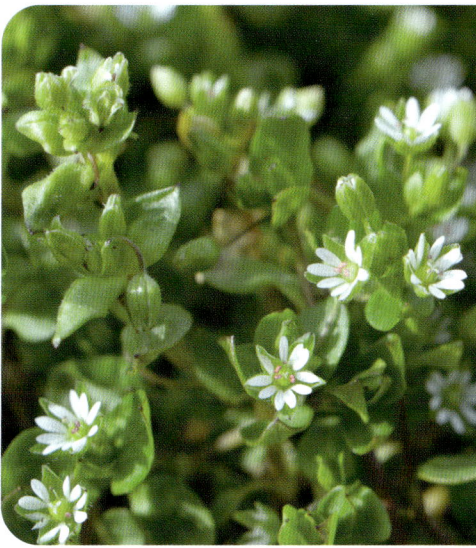

CHICKWEED FAST FACTS

- Plant sprawls across ground, growing erect if supported by other plants
- Fine hairs grow on alternating sides of stem
- Leaves are opposite
- Common in garden beds or disturbed areas
- Harvested year-round, but best gathered in spring
- Stems and leaves can be consumed raw or cooked

PLANTAIN

Plantago major, Plantago lanceolata
Family: Plantaginaceae

Other Names: white man's footprint, doorweed

Parts Used: leaves and seeds

When to Harvest: throughout the year

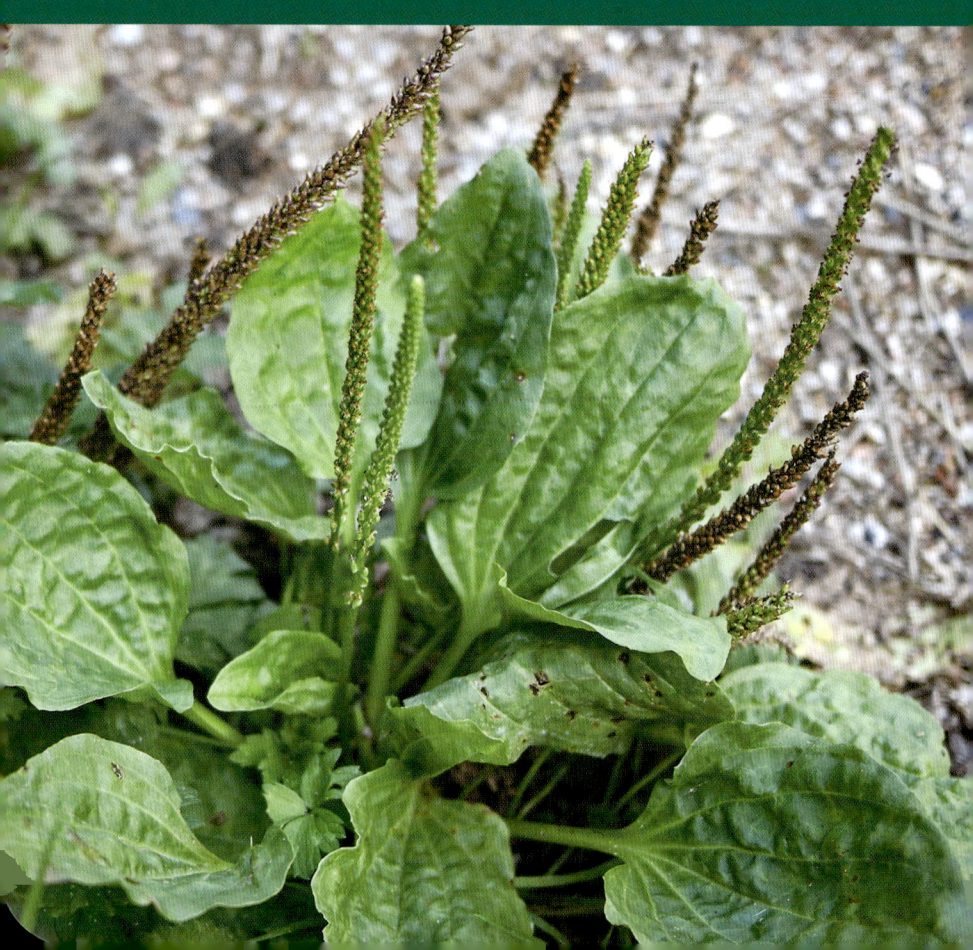

Plantain was one of the first plants I learned to use as a topical herbal medicine. Like chickweed, it showed up in my garden uninvited. Sometimes called "white man's footprint," this plant followed in the footsteps of European settlers hundreds of years ago and has since naturalized throughout the Americas. Its distinctly erect flower and seed heads are an easy identifier. From poultices to tea, plantain is an all-star in the herbal world, and with good reason.

BENEFITS

Nutritive. Rich in vitamins and minerals

Vulnerary. Stimulates wound healing when used topically

Demulcent. Cooling and soothing

IDENTIFICATION

Plantain often grows in large patches; *Plantago major* (which has broad, round leaves) prefers areas that collect rainwater, whereas *P. lanceolata* (which has thinner, longer leaves) tends to grow among grasses and tall plants. All plantain species have basal leaves, stemming from the center of the plant.

When blooming, a tall flower head emerges from the center, with flowers and seeds wrapping around the top segment. *P. major* tends to have larger flowering parts, generally three to five inches in height, while *P. lanceolata*'s are about an inch long. The flowers are white and turn brown after drying. This is a great plant to observe with a loupe, as the flowers are very tiny. The leaves have distinct fibers, running from the stem to the tip, which are typically

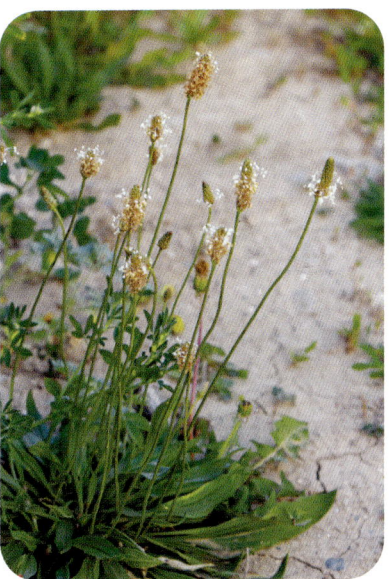

The flowers of *Plantago lanceolata* are white and about an inch long, in contrast to the longer flowers of *P. major* (**opposite**).

removed before eating. Plantain commonly grows in disturbed areas, such as lawns, construction sites, parking lots, and in gravel alongside roads or rivers.

TRADITIONAL USAGE

Plantain is a wonderful topical and internal medicine. Topically, the leaves are crushed into a poultice and applied to ailments such as bee stings, bug bites, and scratches. The cooling, demulcent properties help ease inflammation, itching, and pain. As a vulnerary, it helps promote wound healing and is commonly included in herbal oils and salves.

For internal use, the mildly bitter leaves can be cooked and eaten as a nutritive green rich in vitamin B6, manganese, calcium, beta-carotene, and more. The leaves can also be made into a tea and drunk as a cooling medicine for digestive upset and irritation. Plantain's *mucilage*, a smooth and slimy compound in the leaves (similar to okra's sliminess), is very nourishing and cooling for hot ailments. I like to add dry plantain leaves to tea blends for hydration and cooling in summertime, and even boil the fresh leaves if I don't have the time to dry them.

The seeds are also nutritive, rich in protein, fats, and omega-3s and omega-6s. *P. ovata*, a species of plantain regularly found throughout Asia, is the source of the common supplement called *psyllium husk*. The seeds are considered a bulking laxative and are taken to regulate digestion, like flaxseed or chia seeds. The seeds of other species can be used similarly.

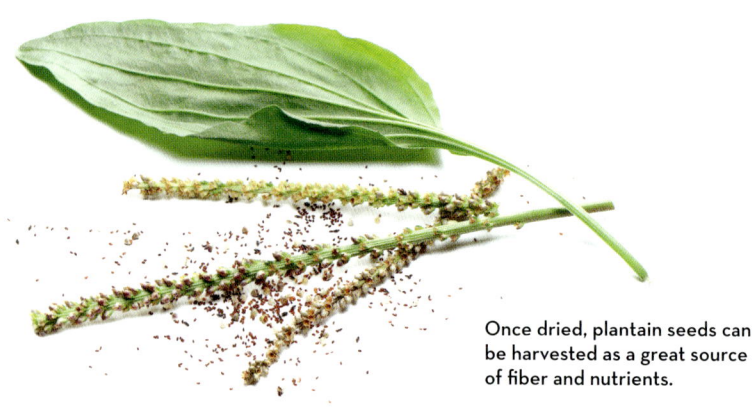

Once dried, plantain seeds can be harvested as a great source of fiber and nutrients.

HARVESTING

Harvest younger plantain leaves, cutting the stem close to the center where they emerge. This plant tends to be abundant and grows throughout the year, so you can harvest it until it dies back in winter. Plantain will bloom multiple times a year if the seed heads are picked. If you're using the seeds, gather the seed heads once they turn brown, dry out, and break easily in your hands when rubbed.

PREPARATION

Plantain is very easy to process without any special equipment. For topical applications, such as for a bug bite, sting, or rash on the skin, simply harvest the plantain leaves and crush them well, applying them to the affected area. This can be done in a mortar and pestle, by chewing the leaves, or by simply ripping them with your hands. Squeeze out the excess water to help the plant break down.

Before cooking or eating the leaves, you'll want to remove the fibers that run through the leaf. Simply cut the stem and find the visible fibers, pulling them slowly to remove. The leaves can also be dried and preserved for oils and teas.

Once the seeds are dried and ready to harvest, cut the flowering stalk, strip the seeds, and lightly roll them between your hands to separate the chaff and

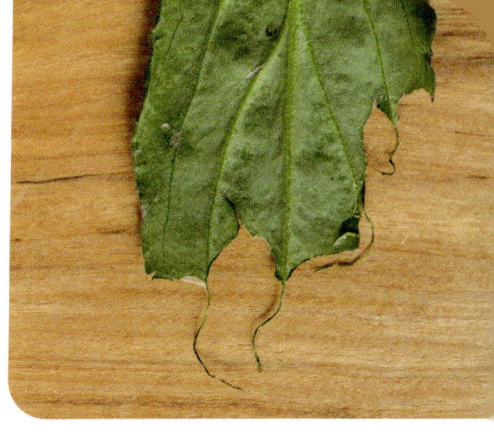

Plantain leaves have tough fibers running through them which are best removed before eating.

shell from the actual seeds. The seeds can be lightly toasted, to "pop" them, and you can eat them in cereals and porridge. They add a nutrient boost to any meal.

PLANTAIN FAST FACTS

- Various varieties; *P. lanceolata* (long, lanceolate leaves) and *P. majora* (broad leaves) are most common
- Grows in garden beds, areas where water gathers, cracks in concrete
- Leaves are basal with flower stem emerging from center
- Occasional purple coloration where leaf touches soil
- Fibers growing through leaf should be removed before eating
- Harvestable year-round

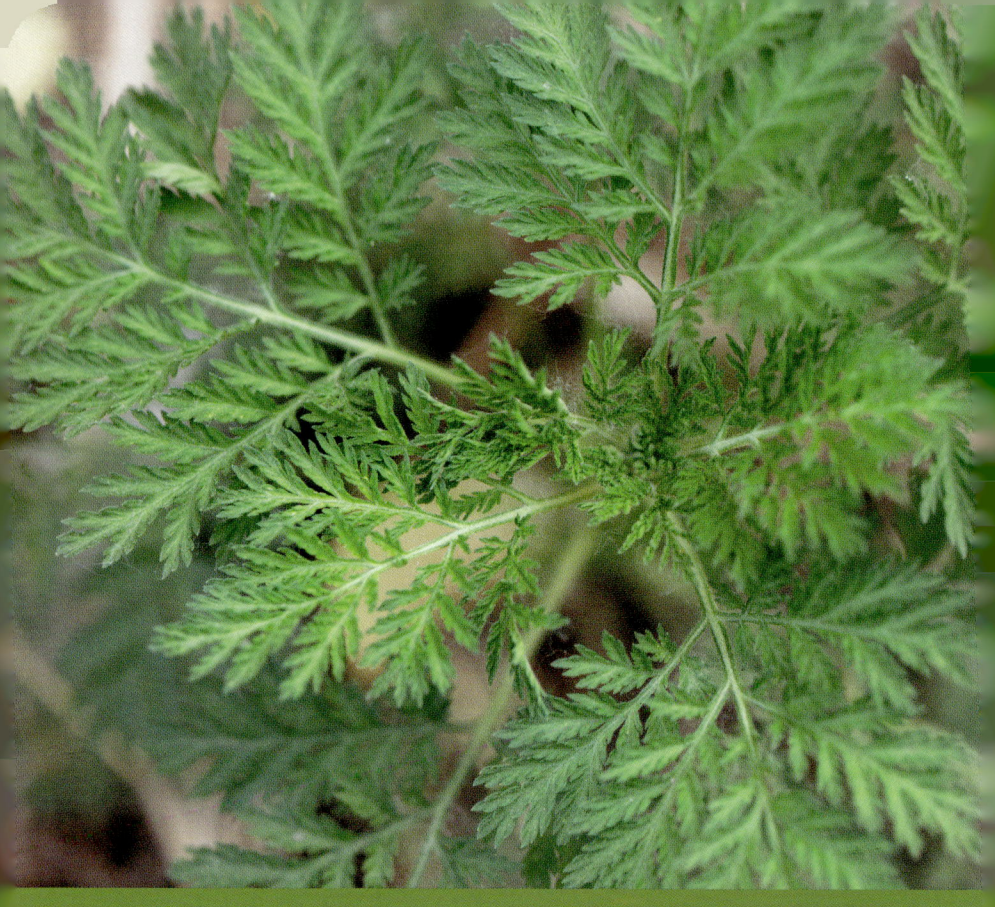

SWEET ANNIE

Artemisia annua
Family: Asteraceae

Other Names: sweet wormwood

Parts Used: flowers and leaves

When to Harvest: late summer and fall

Some say sweet Annie smells like spiced honey, others say it's fruity and floral, but to me it smells like . . . sweet Annie. Sometimes you just can't put a name on it, and you have to leave it with the name it has. Sweet Annie is native to Asia but has become naturalized in North America.

BENEFITS

Antimalarial. Supports the body in combating parasites that cause malaria

Antibacterial. Inhibits bacterial growth

Respiratory tonic. Supports the respiratory system

IDENTIFICATION

Sweet Annie is a tall-growing annual that thrives in disturbed areas such as roadsides and parking lots. Its fine leaves are a vibrant green and pinnately compound, with toothed edges and a smooth texture. The utterly unique aroma is my favorite indicator of sweet Annie, easily experienced by crushing or pulling off a leaf. After you've smelled it once, it will be your best identifying clue. Sweet Annie's flowers are yellow when blooming but appear green after the blooms fade; they look very similar to other flowers from related plants, such as mugwort. The flowers bloom in large clusters at the top of the plant.

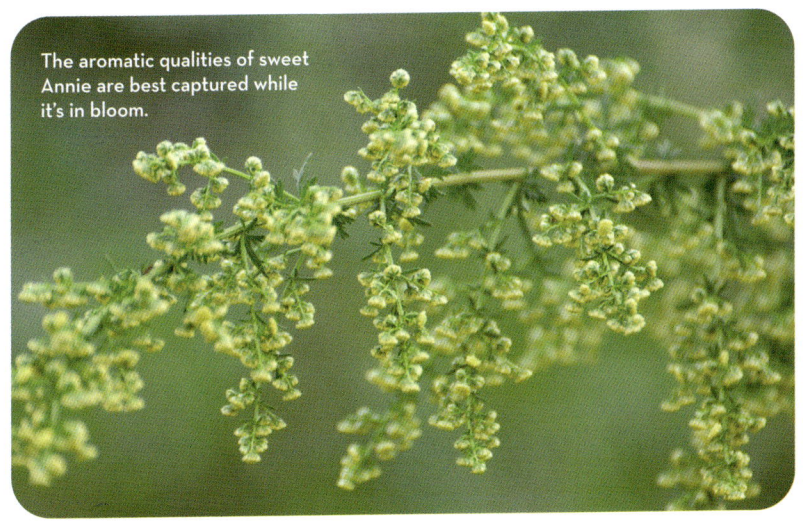

The aromatic qualities of sweet Annie are best captured while it's in bloom.

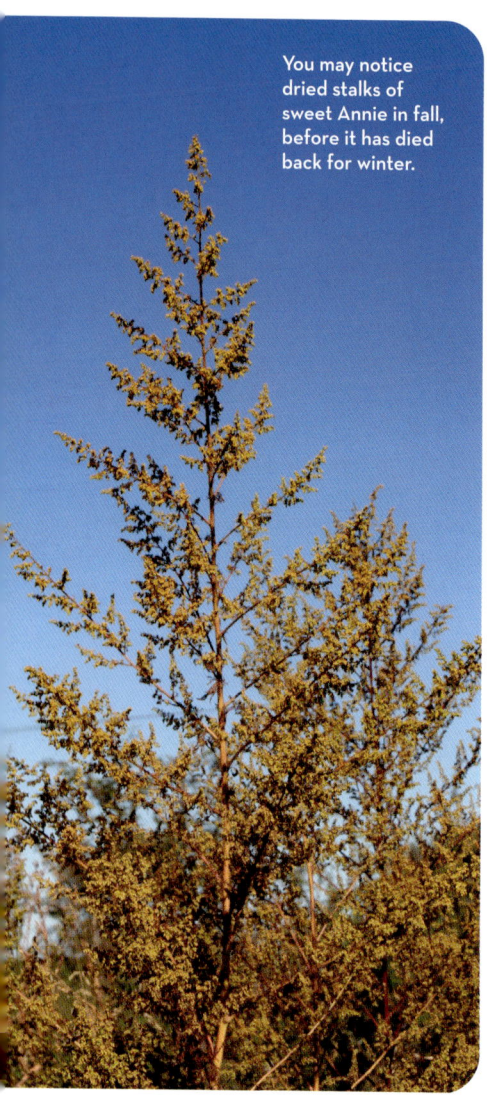

You may notice dried stalks of sweet Annie in fall, before it has died back for winter.

TRADITIONAL USAGE

Sweet Annie has historically been used to address malaria and is still used for this purpose, especially in tropical regions. *Artemisinin* is the active compound responsible for its distinct aroma and its antimalarial qualities. Artemisinin lowers fever and actively fights off the parasite responsible for malaria. It has been used by the pharmaceutical industry in commercial malaria medicines as well.

This plant has an extensive history of use throughout Asia; in traditional Chinese medicine (TCM) it is used for lowering fevers, fighting off infection in the respiratory system, and enhancing circulation in the body with its warming oils. It can be placed around the house to enhance and distribute the aroma, or it can be dried, boiled, and drunk as a medicinal tea. Sweet Annie is excellent in combination with other herbs to support the respiratory system, especially to warm the body during winter.

HARVESTING

Sweet Annie can be harvested before or after flowering, but its aromatic qualities are much more potent once it is in bloom. Sweet Annie is excellent fresh but can also be used dry. If drying, cut the stem a few inches below the flowers and allow them to air-dry. The plant usually begins flowering in late summer and can continue into fall, when it will eventually dry out and die back.

PROCESSING

Sweet Annie tea is a warming aromatic drink that clears the respiratory system and warms the body; both the flowers and the leaves are rich in medicinal compounds. Because it's harvested in late summer and fall, I often keep it dried and preserved for cold and flu season. The fibrous stems don't have as much medicinal quality, so you can strip off the flowers and leaves and discard the stems. Alcohol tinctures extract the aromatic qualities of this plant and help concentrate them to address acute respiratory issues such as congestion and coughing. Vegetable glycerin is also a good option for extracting the medicinal compounds. Sweet Annie glycerin smells incredible!

Avoid If Pregnant

Due to the presence of artemisinin, sweet Annie should not be consumed during pregnancy.

SWEET ANNIE FAST FACTS

- Grows in disturbed areas, sometimes directly in concrete
- Sweet aroma is a good identifier
- Can grow up to six feet tall
- Tiny, yellow flowers when blooming, which dry to a green color
- Small, pinnately compound leaves
- Leaves and flower heads are used medicinally; fibrous stem is less useful

GARLIC MUSTARD

Alliaria petiolata
Family: Brassicaceae

Other Names: poor man's mustard, garlic root

Parts Used: roots, leaves, and flowers

When to Harvest: spring

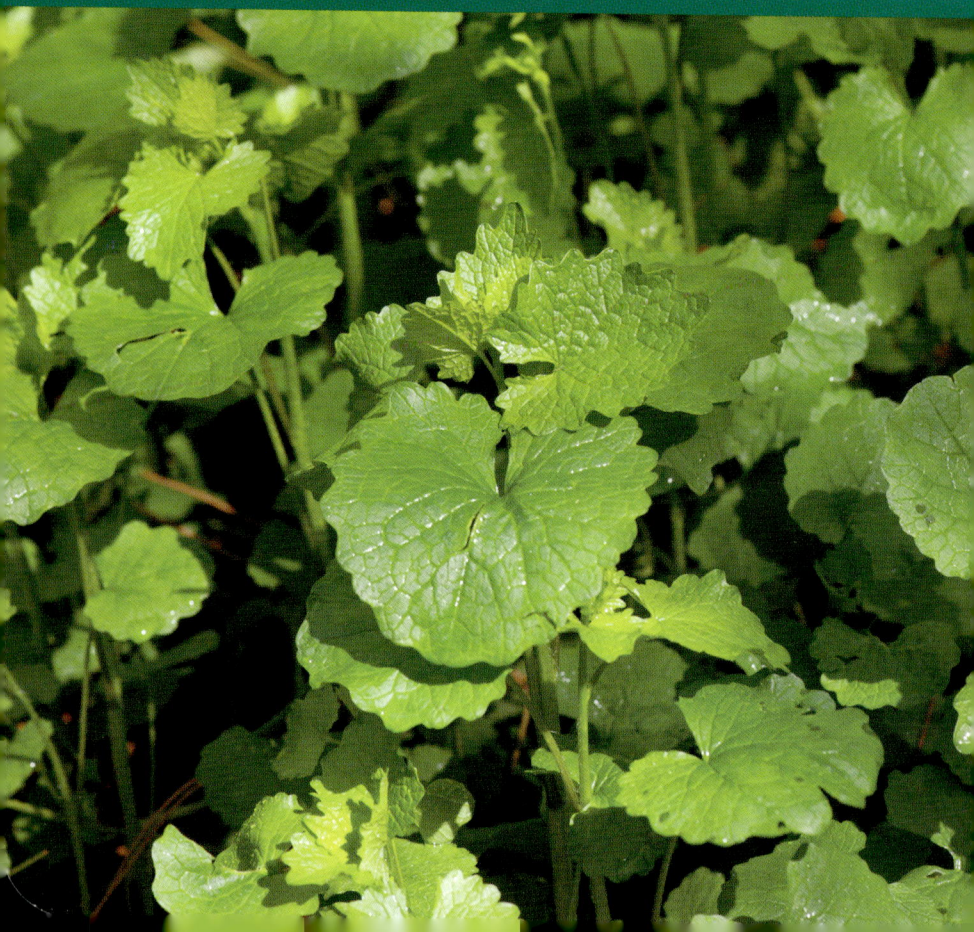

Garlic mustard grows in abundance in the United States, mostly north of Georgia and throughout the Northeast. Originally native to Europe, it reproduces by seed and spreads quickly, producing hundreds of seeds a season. As a biennial it doesn't bloom until its second year, but garlic mustard is still good medicine without its flowering parts. It has a rich, pungent flavor and is full of aromatic oils that are great for health, cooking, and more. You'll see this plant growing at the edges of parking lots and areas with lots of concrete, but its shade tolerance allows it to thrive deep in the forest as well.

BENEFITS

Carminative. Enhances digestion

Decongestant. Reduces nasal congestion

Antibacterial. Inhibits bacterial growth

IDENTIFICATION

During the first year of growth, garlic mustard remains just a few inches tall, growing in a small clump. The kidney-shaped leaves are dark green with scalloped edges. They are hairless, visibly textured, and smell like garlic when crushed.

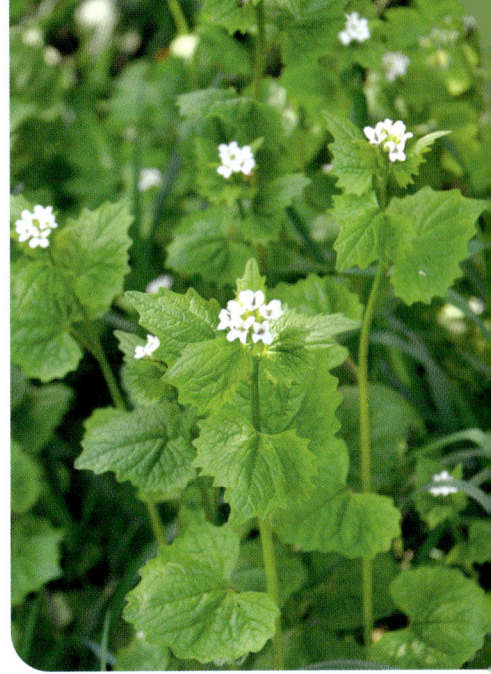

Garlic mustard grows a tall stalk and flowers in its second year of growth.

Garlic mustard blooms during its second year, when it develops a main stalk that grows upward with leaves alternating up the stem. This plant can bloom along any part of the stem, but it flowers most frequently at the very top, with four-petaled white flowers that taste like broccoli when eaten. After blooming, seedpods develop; they are one to two inches long and turn brown and dry out at the end of the season, often remaining on the plant through winter.

TRADITIONAL USAGE

Garlic mustard is used first and foremost as a culinary herb. And like any garlicky, pungent herb, it's excellent for the lungs and digestive system. Garlic mustard leaves and roots can be used as respiratory medicines supporting the body through bronchitis or congestion, and helping cough up mucus. The plant has antibacterial properties that help in combating respiratory infections; it's sometimes used to ease similar issues of the sinus and mouth. You can chew the root for cold sores and oral infections, although your breath will smell for some time after. The leaves can be boiled into tea and drunk as a diuretic to help move fluid through the body and increase urination. As an appetite stimulant, garlic mustard is commonly made into sauces or incorporated into dishes to impart its savory flavor and stimulate digestion.

HARVESTING

I prefer to harvest garlic mustard leaves during the first year, as the flavor is stronger before the plant blooms and goes to seed. Springtime is best, as the first leaves have the most potent flavor. You can also pull the entire plant anytime during the first year and use both the leaves and roots. Since it is so prolific and often suppresses the growth of native plants, harvesting this plant from the root can be beneficial to the overall ecosystem. You can crush the fresh seeds into a flavorful wild mustard paste, or allow them to dry and use them as a garnish or in seasoning blends as you would with other varieties of mustard seed.

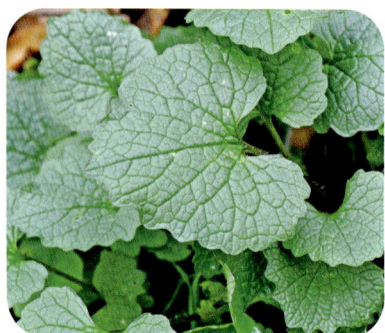 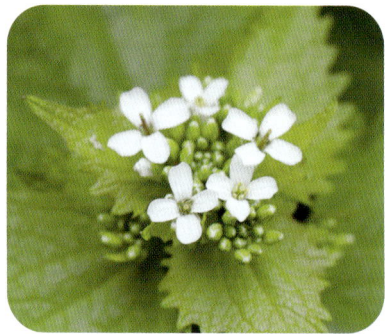

The flavor of garlic mustard is stronger before the plant has flowered.

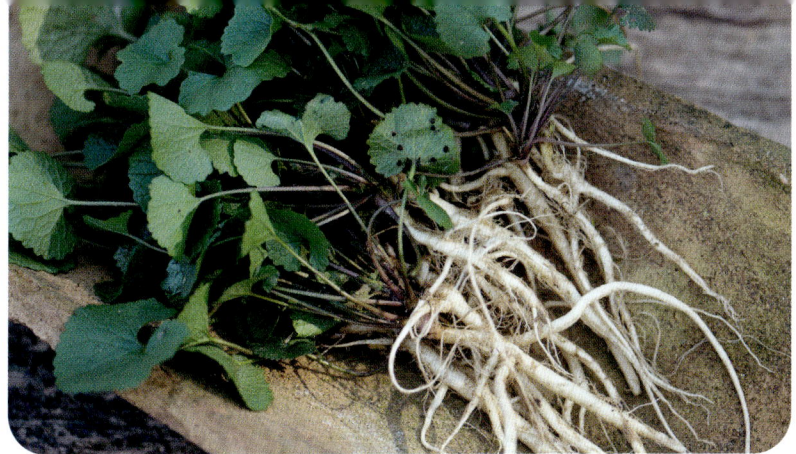

Clean the roots thoroughly (see page 49) before using.

PREPARATION

Garlic mustard leaves are delicious chopped up fresh and added into stews and cooked dishes. (I personally think they're good raw as well; they're just very pungent.) The leaves make a great addition to pesto, chimichurri, or other herbal pastes made with fresh herbs. If you're dealing with sinus congestion or a respiratory issue, try chewing on fresh (clean) roots to benefit from the aromatic compounds. Garlic mustard honey made with fresh roots, leaves, or a combination of both is great as a preventive or treatment for colds, flu-like symptoms, cough, and congestion (see page 240). You can also add garlic mustard to pungent, cleansing medicines such as fire cider to better develop the flavors.

GARLIC MUSTARD FAST FACTS

- Clumps of kidney-shaped leaves with scalloped edges (in the first year)
- Biennial plant, blooming in the second year
- In the second year, it grows a central stalk with alternate leaves; blooms with white flowers
- Grows in shady areas, especially on forest edges
- Emits a strong garlic and mustard-like aroma when crushed
- Entire plant can be used at any stage, raw or cooked

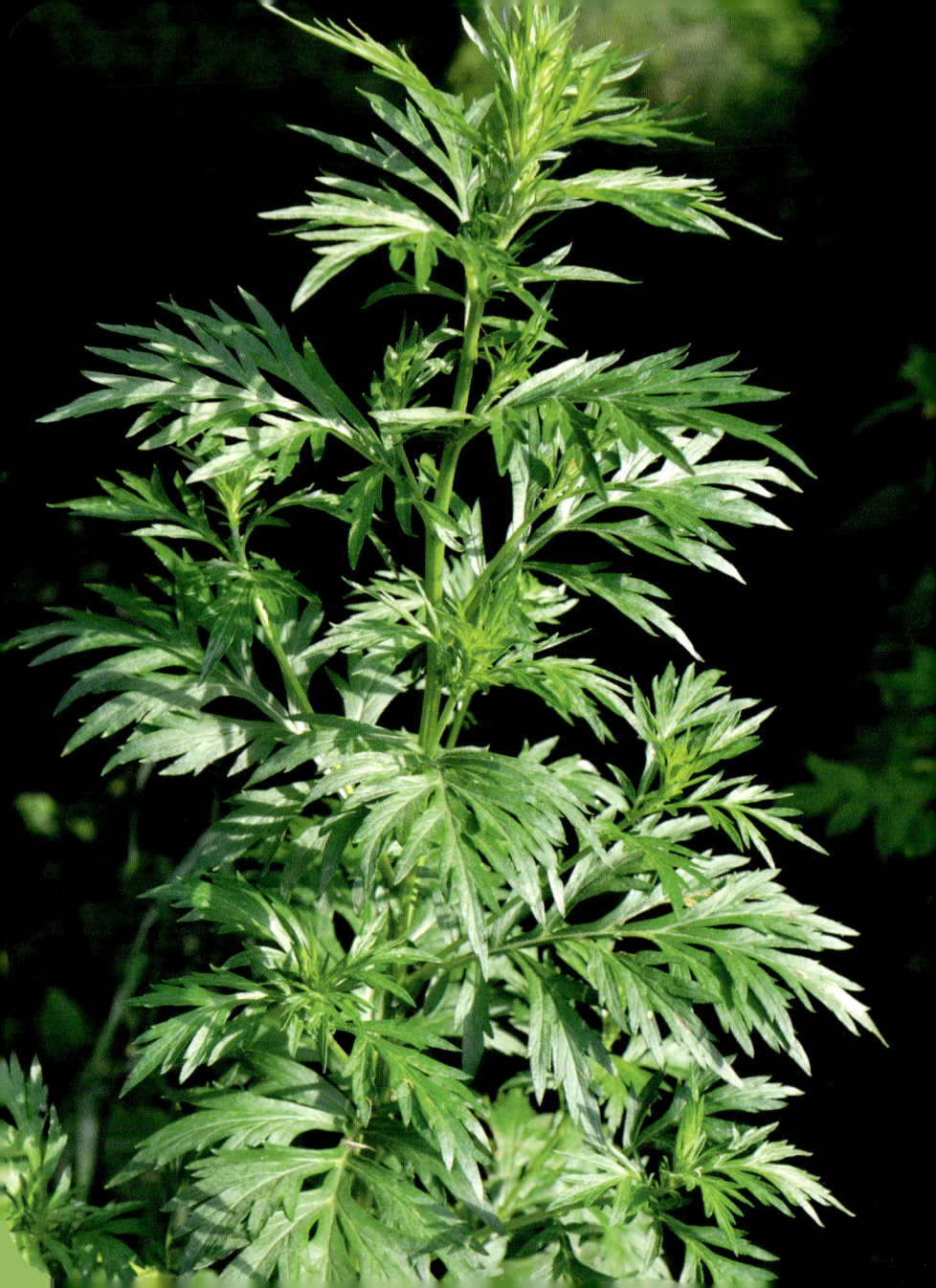

MUGWORT

Artemisia vulgaris
Family: Asteraceae

Other Names: artemisia

Parts Used: leaves and flowers

When to Harvest: spring or midsummer

If you live in the northeastern United States, or anywhere with disturbed areas of concrete and parking lots, you've probably already encountered mugwort. This aromatic friend loves to grow through the cracks on sidewalks in big cities and alongside rivers and industrial areas, where it tolerates both chemicals and intense heat. This plant is native to areas of Europe and Asia but has naturalized throughout most of eastern North America. If you've ever found it growing wild, you'll know it's rare to find one plant on its own—a single mugwort plant can produce a staggering 200,000 seeds per season, making it incredibly abundant.

BENEFITS

Bitter. Stimulates digestion and acts on the liver

Antispasmodic. Eases muscle spasms and cramping

Oneirogen. Stimulates dream activity and lucidity

Anthelmintic. Kills off parasites and worms in the body

Emmenagogue. Increases or stimulates menstruation

IDENTIFICATION

Mugwort's leaves are easy to identify by the silver hairs that grow on the underside, giving them a white color. The top of the leaf is somewhat hairy, but darker in color. The leaves are alternate and lobed. Crushing a leaf will release a warm, pleasant odor that is unique to this plant. Mugwort leaves close up at night, showing their white undersides—a helpful identifier if you're out on a night walk. The new growth tends to point upward. New leaves will have sharper points, while the older leaves have more rounded points and are deeply lobed. The stem often has a purple tone, becoming woodier and green farther down the plant. The flowers grow in clusters at the top of the plant. They are red when freshly blooming, turning silvery green like the rest of the plant as the seeds develop. Mugwort typically grows to be three to five feet tall and even taller once blooming!

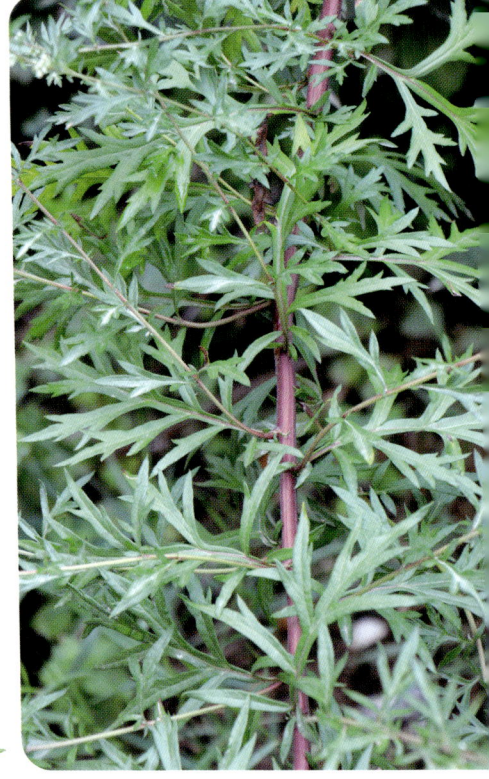

Mugwort leaves have a white or silver underside, while the stems can have a purple tone, becoming greener farther down the stem. Note how the young leaves above are more deeply lobed than the older leaves shown to the left.

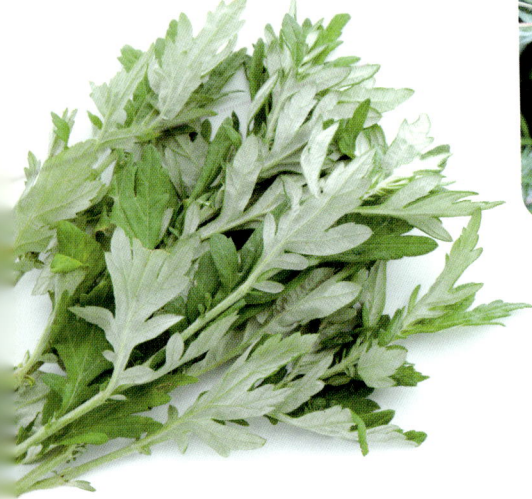

TRADITIONAL USAGE

Mugwort's bitter and aromatic qualities make it a popular ingredient in herbal liquors and bitters throughout Europe, and it has often been used in blends to improve digestion and settle an upset stomach. Mugwort makes an excellent tea for people who hold their anxiety in their stomach, and for easing stomach spasms and cramping after a heavy meal. A tincture can be more approachable than tea, so I keep some mugwort tincture on hand when going out to eat or to offer to guests I cook for. For folks with chronic digestive problems, taking the tea or tincture before and after each meal can aide in regulating digestion.

Mugwort has a history in Europe and Asia as both a physical and a spiritual medicine. It is considered to be protective and is connected to lunar cycles and the dream state. It is an *oneirogen*, a plant that stimulates dream activity and lucidity. Mugwort can be made into a tea, smoked, or even stuffed in pillows to enhance dreams. The plant's lunar connection is reflected in its physical form—the underside of mugwort leaves are a pale, celestial white. As mugwort plants furl their leaves at night, showing the white underleaf to the night sky, it's easy see why so many cultures have connected this plant with the moon.

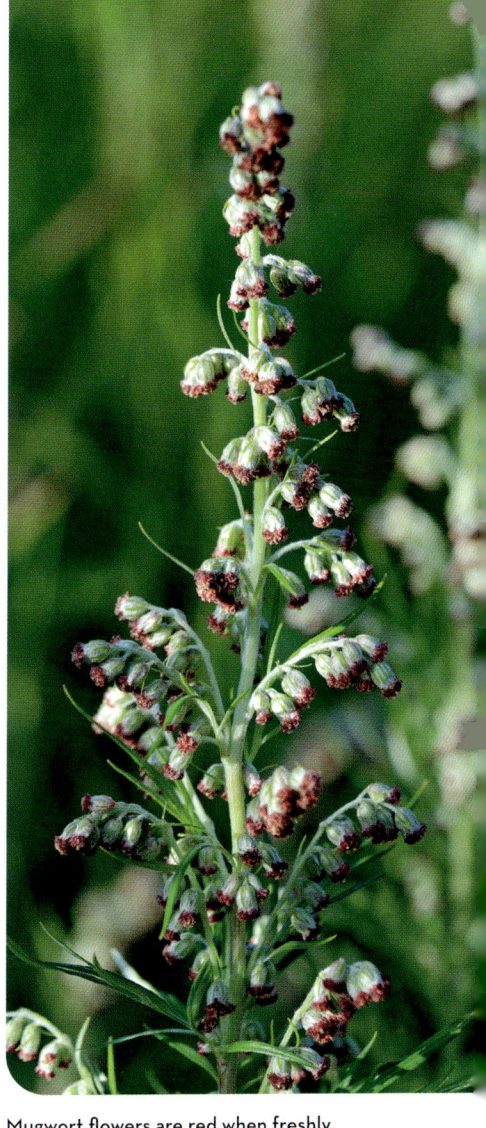

Mugwort flowers are red when freshly blooming; this is when the plant is at its most aromatic.

Avoid If Pregnant

Mugwort should not be consumed during pregnancy or if you are hoping to become pregnant because it can stimulate menstruation.

Mugwort can also be used as an *emmenagogue*, stimulating menstruation, yet another connection to the lunar cycle. It can help regulate a late menstrual cycle, offer uterine support, and aid in postpartum healing.

HARVESTING

The best time of year for harvesting mugwort is either in spring when the first shoots come up or in midsummer when the flowers develop and begin to bloom. Mugwort's aromatic qualities are at their peak when the plant begins to flower. You can harvest both the flower heads and upper leaves or just the upper leaves before the plant blossoms. Doing so will stimulate growth and make the plant bush out horizontally, which creates even more abundance for future harvests. It's important to remember this plant ally can pull up chemicals and heavy metals from the soil, so be mindful of where you're harvesting from.

PREPARATION

Mugwort is a great plant to use fresh or dried in tea making. A simple infusion extracts the bitter and aromatic compounds that support our digestive and nervous systems. Mugwort combines beautifully with vegetable glycerin; the resulting tincture is an easy way to enjoy its digestive benefits. It also works well as an oil or salve, as its aromatic and antispasmodic effects can be used topically for cramps and muscle soreness. There are countless ways to use mugwort, and it's one plant I keep in my medicine cabinet year-round.

MUGWORT FAST FACTS

- Leaves are dark green on top, silver on bottom, with fine white hairs
- Newer leaves sometimes have sharper edges, while older leaves are more roundly lobed
- Leaves curl up at night, showing silver underside
- Warm aromatic quality when crushed
- Best harvested when flowers first emerge or before flowering
- Leaves and flowers harvested, not stem or root

JAPANESE KNOTWEED

Polygonum cuspidatum
Family: Polygonaceae

Other Names: itadori, Japanese bamboo

Parts Used: new shoots and roots

When to Harvest: spring or fall

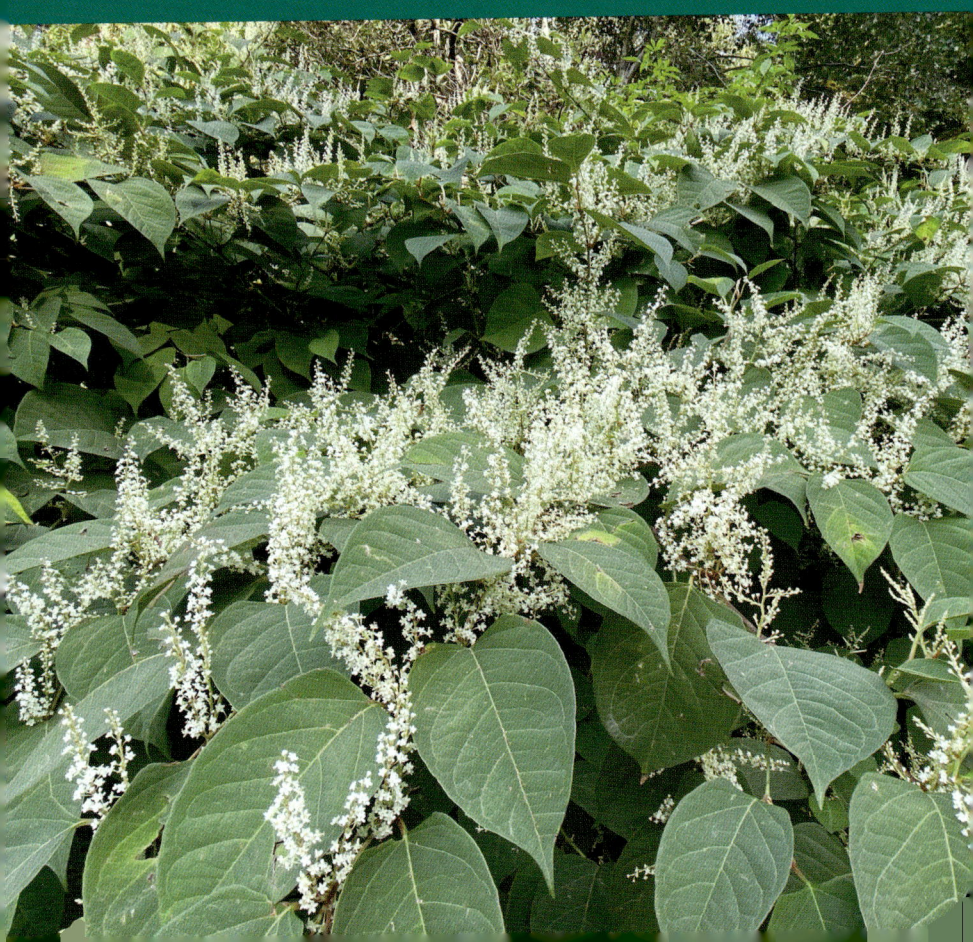

Japanese knotweed is one of my favorite misunderstood herbs. While "invasive" plants do have a detrimental effect on native plants and the environment, demonizing the plants themselves isn't helpful. As herbalists and foragers, we can play the role of mediator, helping people to understand the plant and letting our medicine cabinets and stomachs benefit from its presence. Japanese knotweed is infamous for its ability to spread quickly, send taproots 10 feet down into the soil, and even propagate from just ½ inch of root. A true example of resiliency, Japanese knotweed simply does what it does best—grow. With the right knowledge, we can utilize these excessively abundant plants for healing and food.

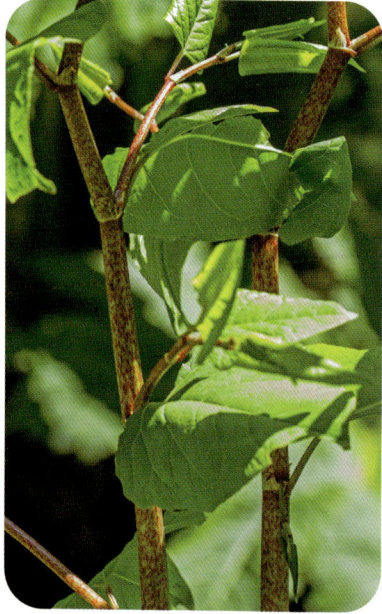

New shoots of Japanese knotweed are speckled with reddish purple spots.

BENEFITS

Alterative. Restores the normal balance and function of the body's systems and organs

Anti-inflammatory. Reduces inflammation in the body

Antiviral. Supports the body in combating viruses

IDENTIFICATION

Japanese knotweed is a perennial herb that emerges in early spring. The first shoots are green with reddish purple spots. They are hollow and resemble bamboo, though the plants aren't related. As the plant develops, the stem grows in a unique zigzag pattern, with dark green, heart-shaped leaves alternating along the length. The white flower clusters are erect, growing along the full length of the stem and blooming in late summer. The plant itself grows between three and six feet tall and tends to form large patches. The roots are brown outside and a rich orange or red inside.

TRADITIONAL USAGE

Japanese knotweed has been used in herbal medicine systems for thousands of years. The roots can be used to detoxify the blood and to fight off respiratory infection, and are considered an overall longevity tonic. Rich in *resveratrol*, a phytochemical found in grapes and red wine that has heart-nourishing properties and helps the body holistically, Japanese knotweed is a general tonic that can be taken regularly to strengthen the heart and cardiovascular system. As a tincture, Japanese knotweed is taken for respiratory ailments, helping ease inflammation in the lungs and fight off viral infections. This plant has even been used in protocols by various herbalists to alleviate symptoms of Lyme disease. The young shoots are also eaten, fresh or cooked, and are often compared to rhubarb in terms of taste.

HARVESTING

When harvesting fresh shoots of Japanese knotweed for food, gather the first emerging shoots when they

Avoid If Pregnant

In high dosages, Japanese knotweed can act as an abortifacient and should be avoided if you are pregnant.

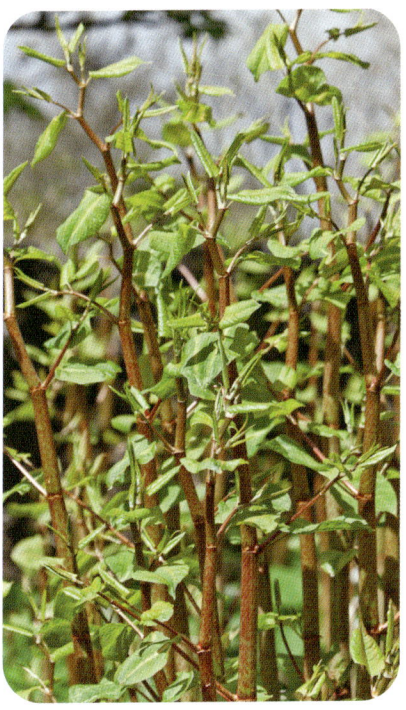

Knotweed shoots are abundant in spring. Since this hardy plant is invasive, you can harvest large amounts to prevent it from spreading further.

Japanese Knotweed

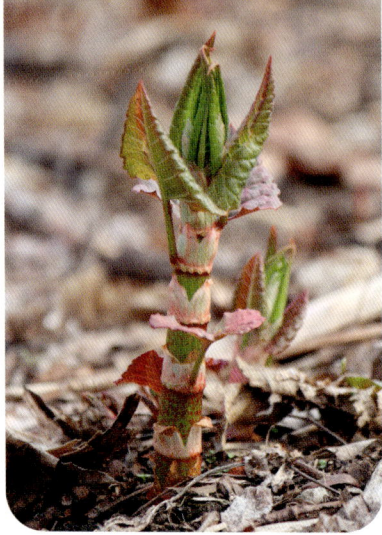

It's best to harvest the shoots when they are tender and flexible, typically when they're about a foot tall or less.

JAPANESE KNOTWEED FAST FACTS

- Stems are hollow and green with reddish spots
- Zigzag growth pattern
- White flowers grow in erect clusters in summer
- Three to six feet tall; loves to grow in disturbed areas
- Grows in large patches that spread via rhizomes
- Shoots can be harvested for food in early spring (eaten raw or cooked); roots for medicinal use in fall

are about a foot tall in early spring. They should bend and make a popping sound when breaking, snapping off easily. Later in the season, the shoots will become tough and fibrous, so it's better to harvest young, fresh plants.

The roots, on the other hand, are best harvested in fall when the plant is beginning to die back. Bring a trowel, a shovel, or maybe an excavator! You'll find large clumps of root just below the surface, but the taproots will grow several feet down and even sideways. Some roots have been found growing 30 feet sideways and 10 feet down! Since this plant has a negative impact on native ecosystems, take as much root as possible when harvesting. Even if you can't remove it all, at least you tried!

PREPARATION

Fresh, new shoots of Japanese knotweed can be eaten raw or cooked and have a distinctly sour flavor. While there are various nutrients in the stalks, the medicinal qualities are more pronounced in the roots. Tincture the roots fresh or dried, or make a decoction with it alone or alongside other herbs. I find tincturing the roots helps address more acute symptoms, as the medicine is more concentrated.

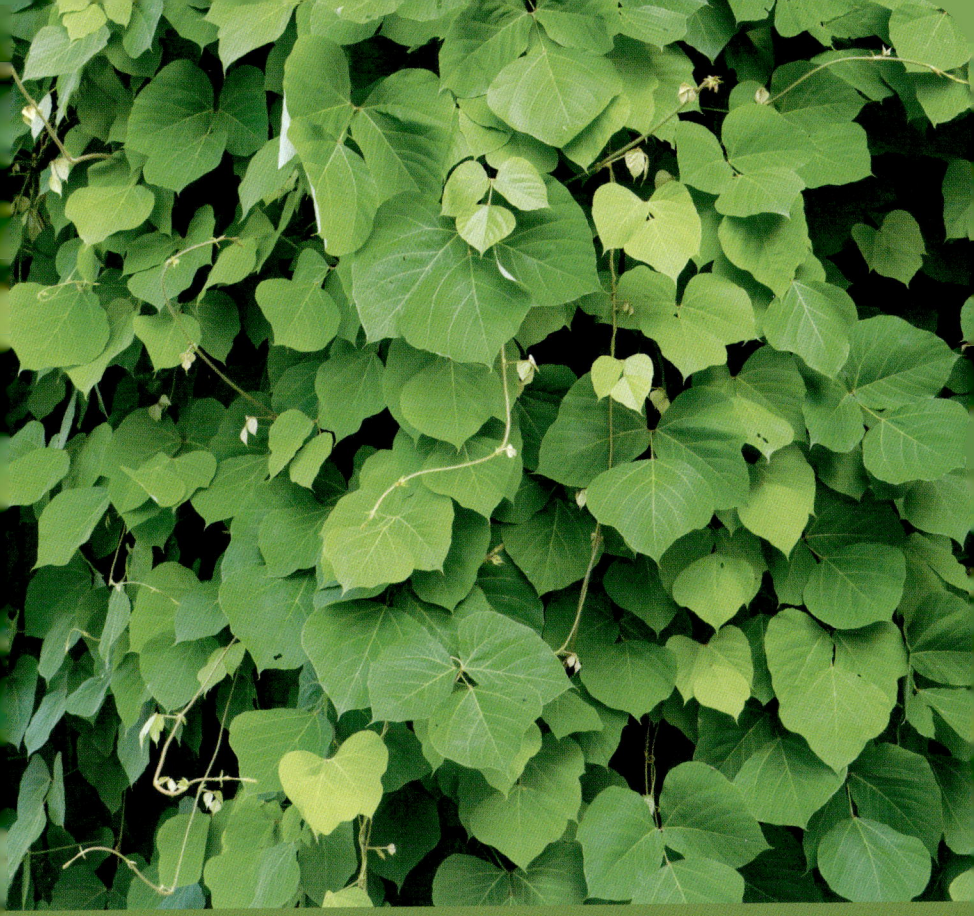

KUDZU

Pueraria montana
Family: Fabaceae

Other Names: the vine that ate the South

Parts Used: leaves, new shoots, roots, and flowers

When to Harvest: spring, summer, and late fall

Sprawling across the landscape of eastern North America, kudzu is another misunderstood plant. Like dandelion and other plants that spread well and aren't native to the ecosystems they thrive in, kudzu covers roadside forests and disturbed areas. Originally native to Japan and parts of eastern Asia, kudzu is an invasive plant in the United States, but it has long been used in cooking, textiles, and medicine.

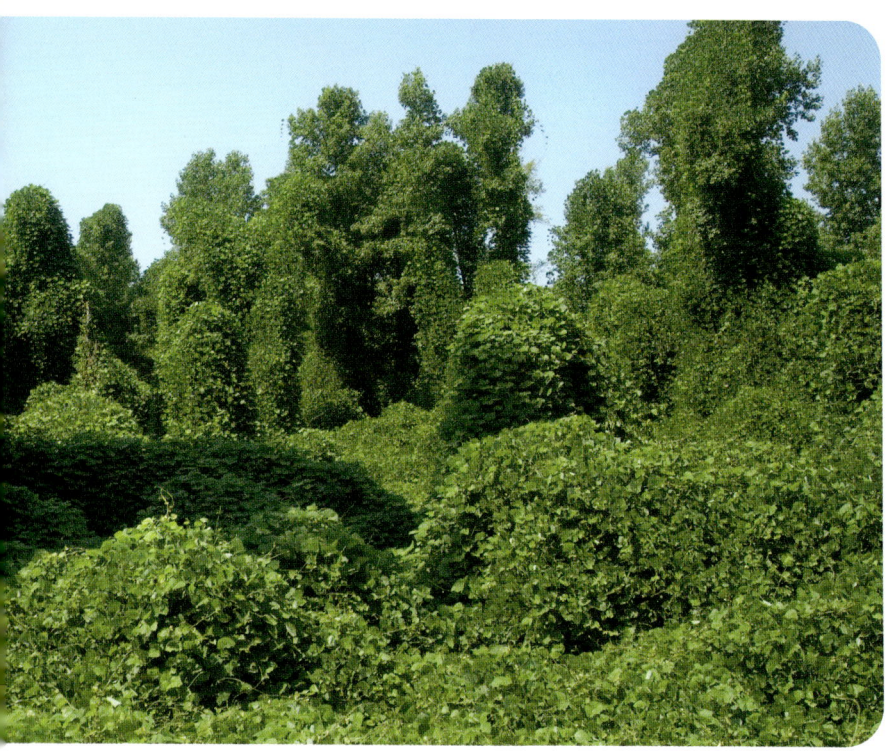

Kudzu can grow to cover everything from trees to telephone poles.

BENEFITS

Cardiovascular tonic. Supports the cardiovascular system

Hypotensive. Lowers blood pressure

Hypoglycemic. Lowers blood sugar

IDENTIFICATION

You'll find kudzu vines covering the ground or growing on trees, often completely smothering them. The leaves are alternate and compound with three large leaflets. The bottom of the leaves and the new vine tips are hairy. The older parts of the plant, farther down the stem, generally appear woodier and don't have hair. The purple flowers are distinctly aromatic and grow in upright clusters, usually blooming in late summer. Aside from these factors, the biggest identification aid is seeing how profusely the vine grows. You might find yourself knee-deep in a kudzu patch, or it could be growing vertically 20 to 30 feet into trees!

TRADITIONAL USAGE

Kudzu has a long tradition of use in TCM and Japanese herbalism. It's thought to address a myriad of ailments, including alcohol intoxication, high blood pressure, menstrual cramps, fever, and diabetes, among other things.

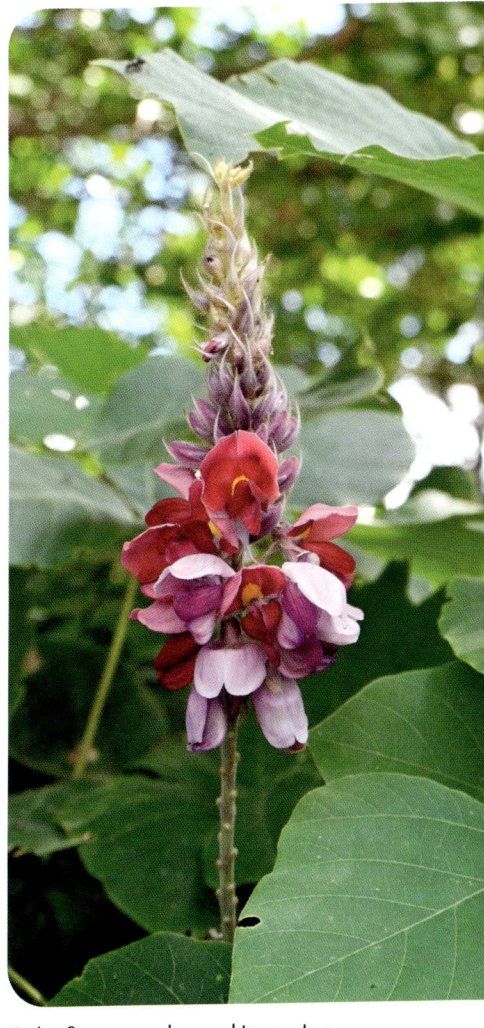

Kudzu flowers can be used to create a mildly sweet tea, with a cooling energy.

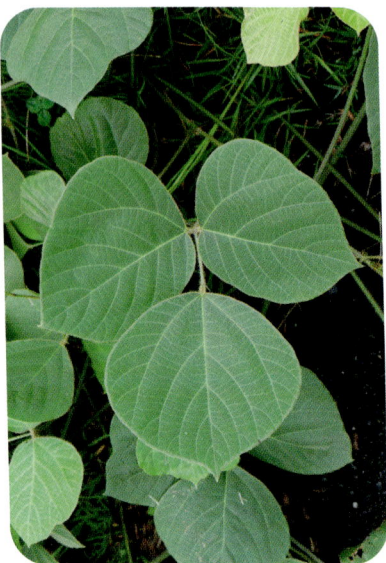

Look for tender new growth when harvesting kudzu leaves.

In the intricate system of TCM, the energy of this plant is considered to be cooling and sweet. Though I'm not a TCM practitioner, I've found this to be true, as drinking a decoction of kudzu displays its mildly sweet, nutritive flavor.

Kudzu can be used as a regulating tonic for blood sugar and blood pressure levels, to support the respiratory system, and for hangover symptoms. Kudzu root works well alongside other plants such as mullein (page 95), for the lungs, or reishi (page 185), as a supporting element. Kudzu root is traditionally taken in capsules or tea, though I often make a decoction of the dried root pieces, or I tincture it for a more acute effect.

HARVESTING

Kudzu flowers can be harvested when fully in bloom in summer; simply pluck the entire cluster of flowers so it doesn't develop seedpods. These seedpods and the seeds within them are inedible and allow the plant to spread, so it's nice to pick the flowers instead! When harvesting the leaves and shoots, new growth is best, so plan to harvest them in spring or summer when they are the most tender.

Kudzu roots tend to grow very deep and can be tricky to harvest without the right tools. Bring both a large shovel and trowel; the first for digging deep enough to access the roots, and the second to allow more precision and to avoid breaking the roots. Roots can be dug in late fall as the plant starts to die back; just follow the vines back to where they originated. The vines propagate by growing small roots wherever they touch the soil, so it can be tricky to find the plant's primary root system. You can pull the vine as you go until you find the main root (which can take some time, so clear your calendar!).

PREPARATION

The roots have the strongest medicinal benefits. Once harvested, scrub them well, then chop them finely and dry them for preservation. After drying, you can use kudzu root herbal decoctions for respiratory ailments, blood sugar regulation, and as a general tonic. To use the roots fresh, tincture them in a medium- to high-proof alcohol (40 to 70 percent). Instead of chopping, you can grate the root to allow more surface area for extraction. The leaves and fresh shoots can be briefly steamed or boiled and eaten, and the flowers create an aromatic and mildly sweet tea when made into an infusion. Remember, the seeds are not edible.

KUDZU FAST FACTS

- Vines usually cover the ground or tree they're growing on
- Leaves alternate on stem, which is fuzzy when new and woody when mature
- Leaves are compound with three leaflets
- Upright purple flower clusters, aromatic when blooming in summer
- Roots best harvested in fall when leaves begin to die back
- Be cautious of where you're harvesting; many people spray herbicides on this plant

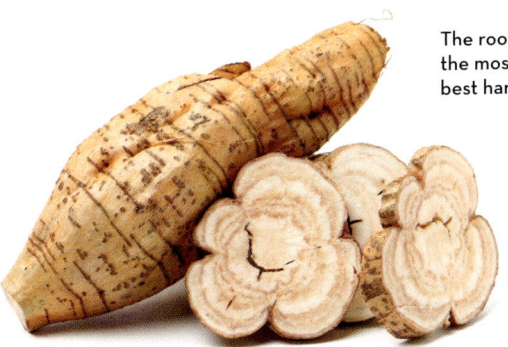

The roots of the kudzu plant have the most medicinal value and are best harvested in late fall.

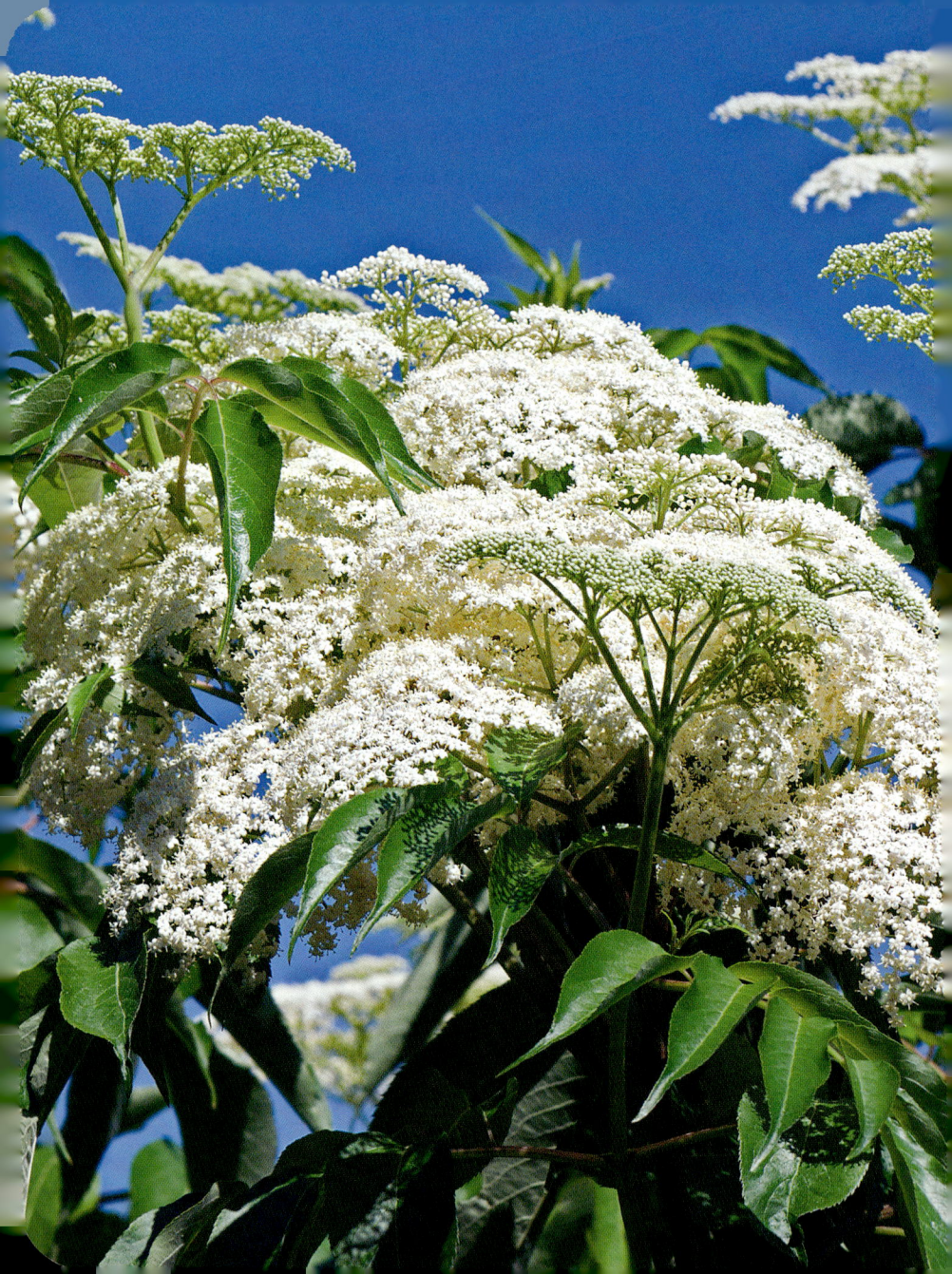

CHAPTER 5

WILD HERBS
from the Field

The plants in this chapter grow abundantly in sunny fields—but like many of our plant allies, they're resourceful and can also grow in a myriad of unexpected places. Whether you live deep in a forest or in a bustling city, foraging will help you pay more attention to the nature that surrounds you, the environment where plant species thrive, and how resilient and dynamic our plant allies really are.

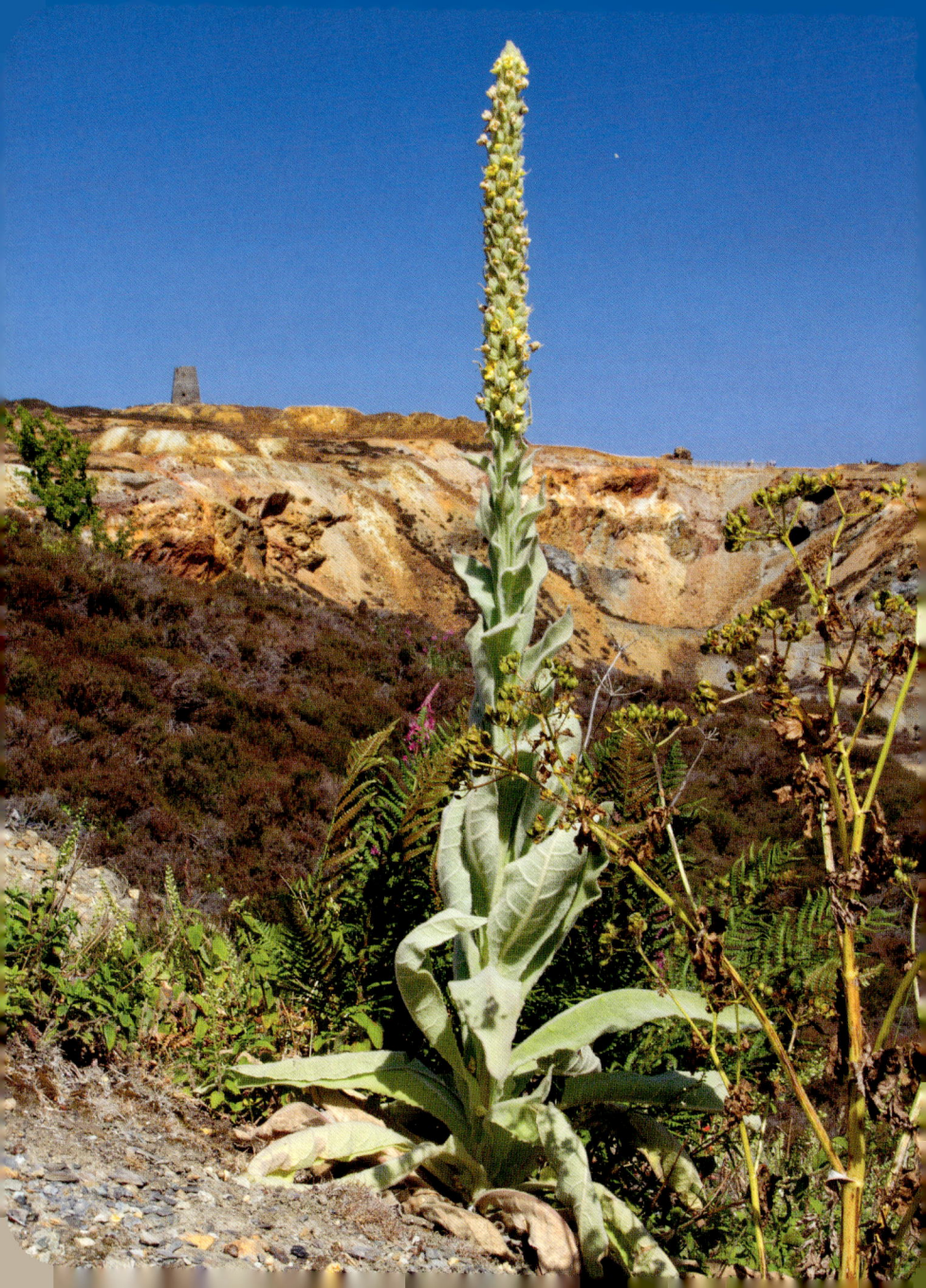

MULLEIN

Verbascum thapsus
Family: Scrophulariaceae

Other Names: candlewick plant, torches

Parts Used: leaves and flowers

When to Harvest: summer

This fuzzy, soothing plant is commonly used to ease various respiratory ailments and grows abundantly throughout the Americas. Although originally native to Asia, North Africa, and Europe, mullein has naturalized in North America. A resilient medicine found in disturbed areas such as roadsides and paved spaces, mullein has been used medicinally throughout its native regions. Mullein is easy to find and dries well; it's become a staple of my apothecary.

BENEFITS

Demulcent. Soothes and coats the throat and respiratory system

Expectorant. Aids in clearing mucus from the chest

IDENTIFICATION

Mullein grows from a basal rosette, with all leaves growing from the center. Its leaves are oblong and densely hairy, growing up to a foot long. Sometimes confused with lamb's ears, mullein is a green color complemented by a silvery sheen from the fine hairs. In contrast, lamb's ears has much smaller leaves and distinctly white hairs. During its second year, a large flowering stem will emerge from the

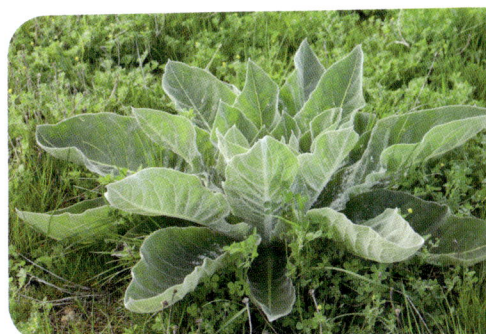

In its first year, mullein grows as a basal rosette without a flower stalk.

center of the mullein plant. The stems can reach up to seven feet tall in some species, with bright yellow flowers whorled around the flower head and alternating leaves toward the base of the stem.

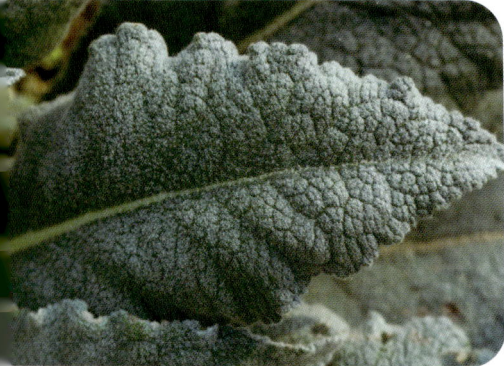

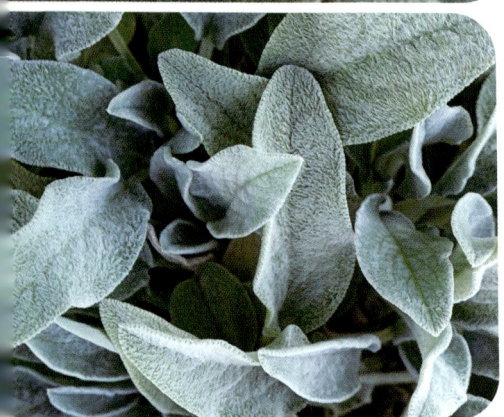

Mullein leaves (top image) are green and grow up to a foot in size, whereas lamb's ears foliage (bottom image) has whiter coloring and much smaller leaves.

TRADITIONAL USAGE

Mullein has long been known as a powerful respiratory tonic. As a demulcent, its soothing and cooling properties help ease the inflammation and irritation that come with a cough. The leaves can be boiled to make a tea to aid in coughing up mucus and phlegm, heal the respiratory tract, and relieve irritation from dry coughs. Mullein has also been smoked to help clear the lungs, but since any sort of smoke irritates the respiratory tract, I wouldn't recommend it. Mullein flowers are often infused into oil, warmed, and dropped in the ears to help earaches and inflammation. The oil can be used topically as a cooling anti-inflammatory for irritation of the skin.

HARVESTING

Collect mullein leaves a month or two after they've first emerged, selecting leaves from the rosette. Cut the stems close to the center to stimulate new leaf growth.

As a biennial, mullein will only bloom in its second year of growth; if you're hoping to harvest the flowers, you'll need an older plant. It will bloom throughout the summer of its second year, and the flowers can be easily plucked off. It's best to have a jar or basket to gather the flowers so they don't get crushed in transport.

PREPARATION

Mullein leaves dry very easily, so I often harvest them in summer and dry them for use in fall and winter. Mullein is a great addition to herbal cough syrups, as the soothing, demulcent quality helps the respiratory system. A simple tea will suffice, but tinctures can also be made to provide higher doses for acute ailments.

Mullein isn't very aromatic, but it can complement aromatic herbs such as sweet Annie (page 70) or bee balm (page 160), which are also used for respiratory support, to help clear congestion, and to warm the chest. Once dried, the flowers can be used infused in oil, whether for soothing irritated skin or helping earaches.

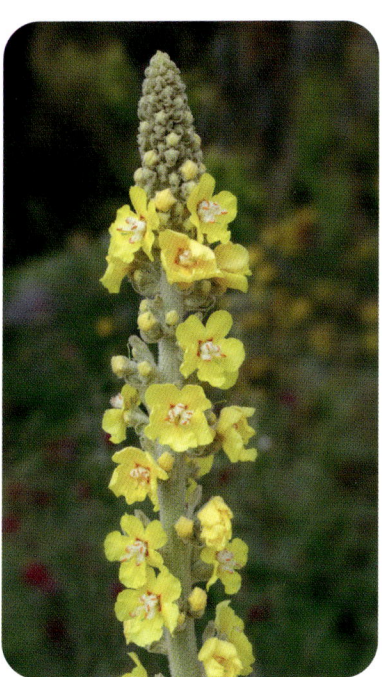

Mullein flowers can be dried and infused into oil to create a topical remedy.

MULLEIN FAST FACTS

- Oblong leaves are basal with fine hairs across surface
- A biennial plant, blooming in the second year
- Produces one tall flower stalk with leaves alternating up stem and yellow flowers whorling around seed head
- Tall stalks of dried flower heads sometimes remain from previous year and are a good indicator of where it may be growing
- Prefers to grow on rocky hillsides and disturbed areas
- Mullein's leaf hairs cannot be bent or pressed down when wet, unlike those of lamb's ears, which will look like wavy hair when wet

VIOLET

Viola odorata, Viola sororia
Family: Violaceae

Other Names: English violet, sweet violet

Parts Used: flowers and leaves

When to Harvest: early spring and summer

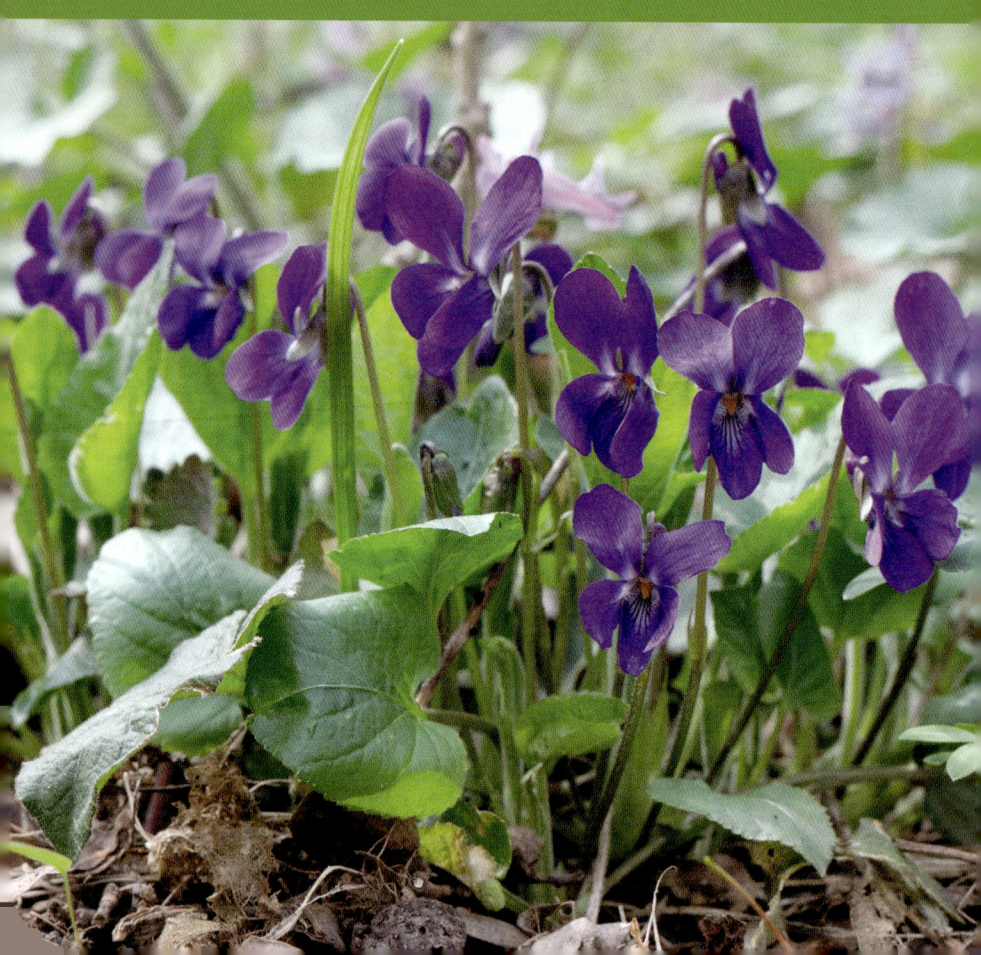

A common spring ephemeral, violets bloom early in the season, signifying that warmer weather is on its way. The leaves and flowers are both used as food and medicine. The flowers make for a bright, colorful addition to a meal. For medicinal purposes, the leaves are more potent than the flowers, though I can never resist picking a few flowers when I walk across a field full of their blooms. Violet tends to like open spaces such as yards or disturbed areas. It typically grows just a few inches tall and avoids competing with taller plants, so it's often easy to spot.

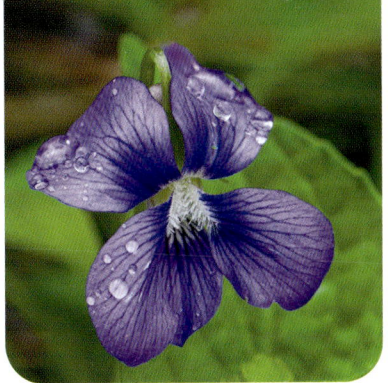

V. odorata is originally from Europe and always blooms purple.

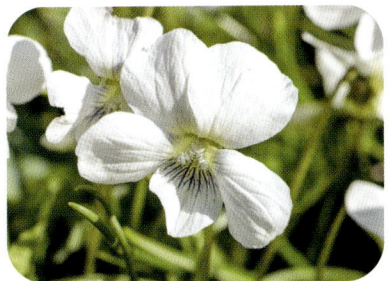

V. sororia can produce purple flowers as well as white blooms.

BENEFITS

Demulcent. Cooling and soothing

Anti-inflammatory. Eases inflammation

Lymphatic. Stimulates lymphatic drainage

IDENTIFICATION

Viola odorata, the species native to Europe but naturalized in North America, has purple flowers that grow on a stem emerging directly from underground. *V. sororia* is the violet species native to North America; the two species are virtually identical and can be used interchangeably. However, *V. sororia* can also produce white flowers with purple streaks emerging from the center, in addition to the more common purple blooms streaked with white at the center. Violet's leaves are basal and heart shaped with rounded lobes. The flower stem emerges upward and then droops forward before blooming. The flowers themselves have five petals.

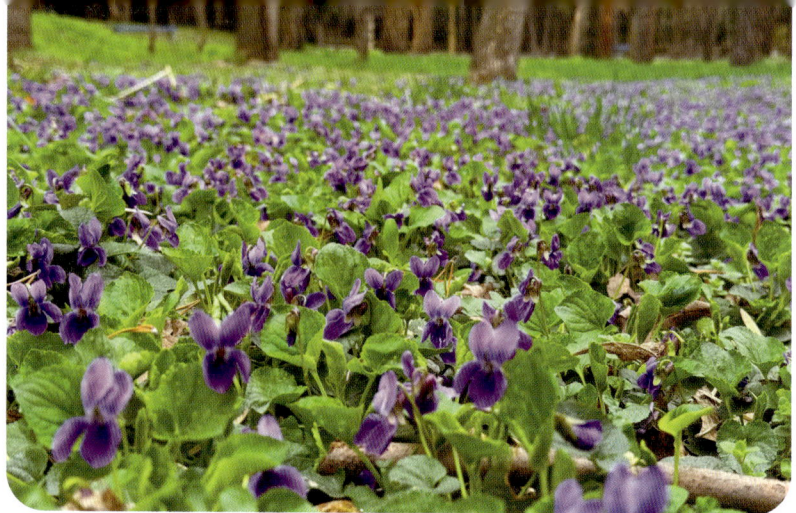

Violets can often be found blooming in fields, meadows, and lawns in spring.

TRADITIONAL USAGE

Violet flowers and leaves have been used in herbal medicine throughout Europe and Asia. One of the main benefits of this plant is its demulcent, cooling action. Rich in mucilage, the flowers and especially the leaves soothe irritation and soreness in the respiratory system and stomach. It's best used as a tea or by eating the leaves and flowers directly. Topically, violet holds these same cooling, demulcent qualities, helping calm hot ailments such as rash, eczema, psoriasis, and even sunburn. As an anti-inflammatory, violet supports many of the same issues, cooling hot conditions such as fever, inflammation in the stomach, and swelling in the throat from infection.

As a lymphatic, violet helps facilitate lymph drainage. Like other springtime plants, such as cleavers (page 58), it helps shake off winter stagnancy. In addition to tea, violet is traditionally used to make an oil or salve that can be massaged into the body, specifically the lymph nodes and breasts. When applied to the breasts, this soothing oil can ease inflammation and swelling and facilitate the drainage of the lymphatic system.

HARVESTING

Violet is best harvested in spring and summer. The flowers die back at the beginning of summer, but the leaves remain usable. Violet likes to grow in large patches, so you can pick a few leaves from each plant to ensure there's enough for other humans and creatures. The flowers tend to have a very short shelf life, so plan to use them the same day. The leaves dry well and can be saved for later use. If you pull the entire plant up, just make sure to cut off the root, as it's considered inedible and won't serve any medicinal purposes.

PROCESSING

Violet flowers are a great addition to salads and pastries; they're edible raw or cooked. I personally prefer them raw as they have more flavor and color. They lend vibrant color to drinks or vinegars, and some folks like to dry them for later use. I find violet most effective when eaten raw or dried and drunk as tea, as opposed to tincturing. Violet leaves and flowers can be used to make an oil. If making into an oil, dry the leaves to keep the water content low, especially considering violet's mucilaginous consistency. Both leaves and flowers dry relatively quickly and easily.

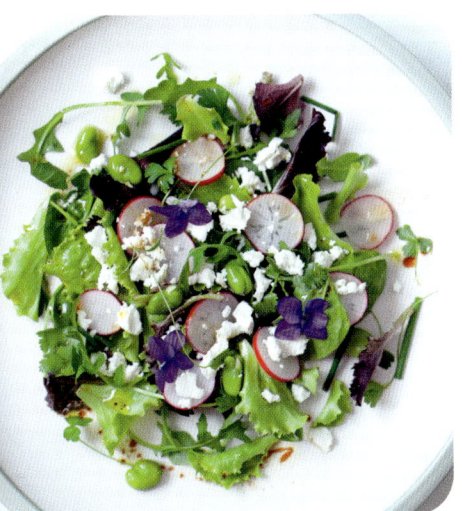

Violet flowers are a colorful addition to spring salads. Just be sure to harvest plants that haven't been sprayed with herbicides.

VIOLET FAST FACTS

- Rounded leaves emerging directly from soil
- Flower emerges from ground on a stem that curls downward
- Flowers have five petals with contrasting streaks inside
- *V. odorata* blooms purple, but native North American species can be white
- This plant likes to grow in disturbed areas or garden beds; it spreads quickly and is often found in large patches
- Blooms in spring, sometimes blooming again in fall during similar temperatures

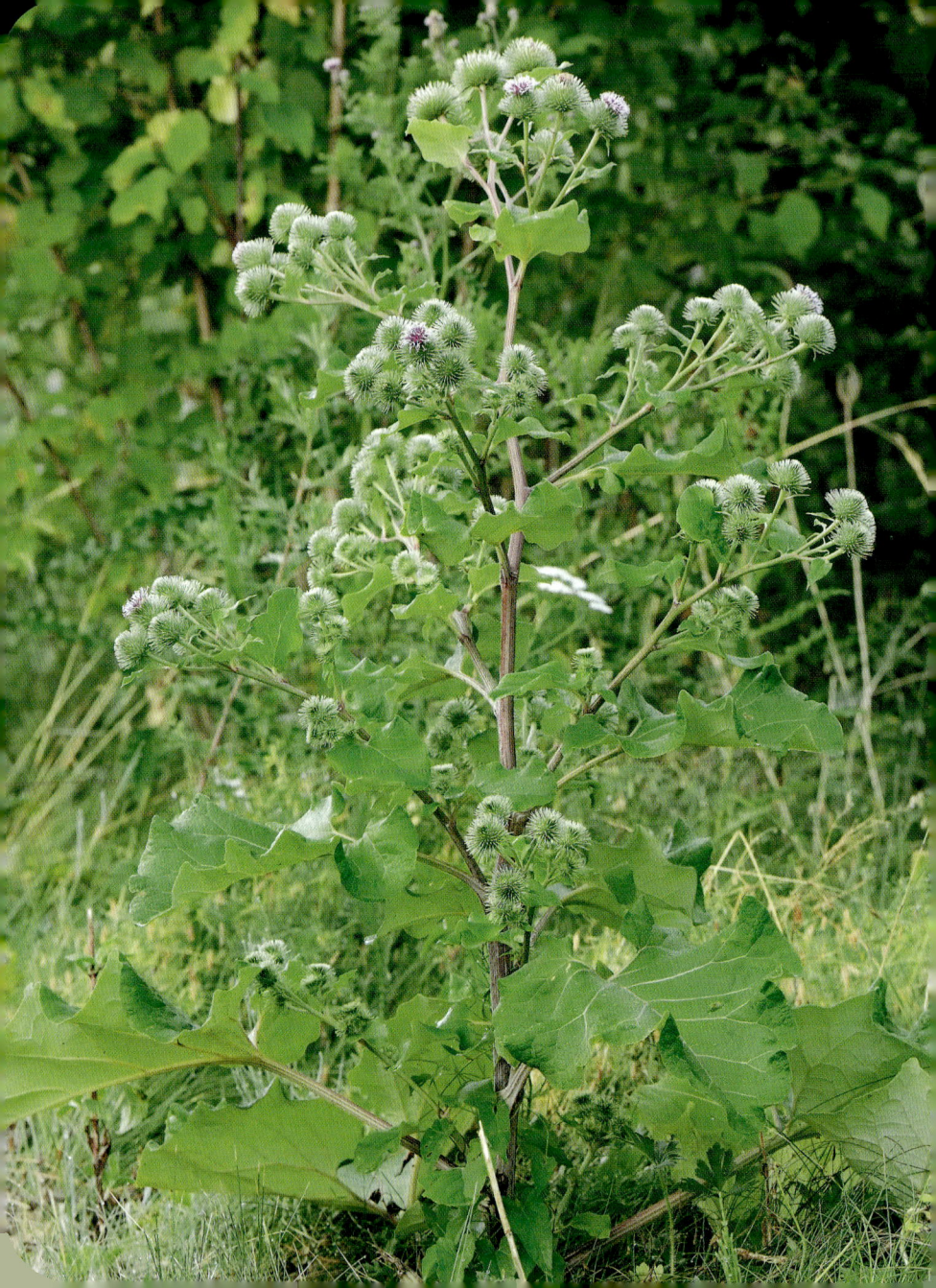

BURDOCK

Arctium lappa
Family: Asteraceae

Other Names: gobō, beggar's buttons

Parts Used: leaves, roots, and seeds

When to Harvest: spring and fall

Burdock is a perfect example of food as medicine. It's easily found at Asian markets and used in many recipes. While the roots are the most commonly used part of the plant, the leaves and seeds share similar qualities and can be used as both food and medicine.

BENEFITS

Alterative. Restores the normal balance and function of the body's systems and organs

Nutritive. Rich in vitamins and minerals

Diuretic. Helps the body eliminate excess water through increased urination

Prebiotic. Supports the gut by nourishing helpful bacteria

IDENTIFICATION

Burdock is a biennial herb that is easy to identify during both its first and its second year. In spring, burdock's basal leaves emerge from a single point. The leaves are longer than they are wide, with a gently rounded triangular shape. They have a waxy top and fuzzy bottom and can grow more than a foot the first year. The second year, the plant sends up its flowering stem with leaves alternating along the length. Burdock's flower heads emerge in clusters at the top of the plant and are pink, somewhat similar to thistle. However, the only prickly part of burdock is the flower heads and burs, whereas thistles have spikes on the entire plant. You may notice skeletons of burdock plants in late fall. The burs will fall off easily—perhaps a little too easily, as they latch onto clothing, shoes, and even hair.

TRADITIONAL USAGE

The entire burdock plant can be used medicinally, though I primarily focus on the roots. Burdock root is rich in *inulin*, a prebiotic fiber that passes through our digestive tract and nourishes our gut flora. Eating the roots raw or cooked is the best way to enjoy burdock's gut-health benefits. Inulin-rich foods can cause gas in some people, so keep that in mind!

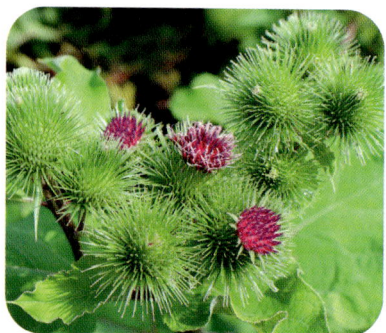

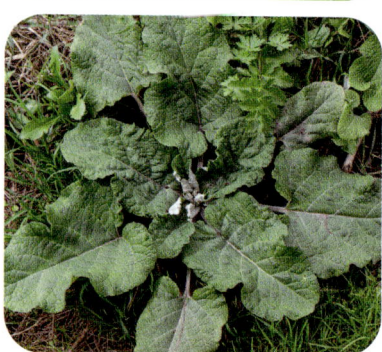

In its first year, burdock grows as a basal rosette without any flowers.

Burdock root is also a powerful alterative and diuretic, helping move the blood and increase urination and the flow of water in the body. It has been used for issues such as edema and is considered a blood cleanser in various traditional medical systems, removing impurities and toxins in the blood.

Burdock is also a great nutritive herb, rich in vitamins and trace minerals such as vitamin B6, manganese, folate, and phosphorus. The nutritive effects of burdock are best absorbed through eating, whereas the alterative and diuretic effects are best demonstrated through tinctures. Alternatively, a decoction will capture all three aspects. Burdock leaves and seeds have much the same impact as the roots and can be made into tea or tinctured.

Both the roots and the seeds are thought to be beneficial for skin issues such as eczema and psoriasis if taken over a long period of time.

HARVESTING

Burdock blooms the second year of its life. Harvest the taproot once the flowers dry and the stem dies, but avoid harvesting late in winter, when roots become overly fibrous. You can harvest the roots at the end of the first year, but they tend to be much smaller than they would be the second year. Gather

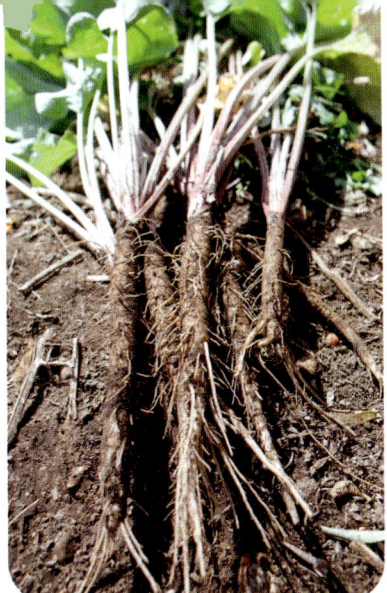

Burdock roots are used both medicinally and as a key ingredient in many Chinese and Japanese recipes.

PREPARATION

Eating burdock roots is one of the best ways to benefit from their medicine. Many Japanese and Chinese recipes include the thinly sliced roots; they can be eaten raw or cooked. For concentrated medicinal usage, try a strong decoction of boiled roots along with leaves if you have them. The leaves aren't as potent as the roots, so I often reserve them for tea instead of tincturing them in alcohol. Burdock's seeds can be crushed and tinctured to extract their medicinal qualities. However, they don't taste the best on their own, as I've learned the hard way.

the leaves in early spring while they are still tender, regardless of how old the plant is.

The seeds can be harvested once the flower heads dry. Wear some thick gloves, as the burs can be difficult to open and will get stuck in your skin! Cutting the dried seedpods, stepping on them, and rolling them under your foot helps get the seeds out. Then collect them and separate the burs and flower parts from the seeds. Sprinkle some of the seeds onto the ground if you want another harvest in future years.

BURDOCK FAST FACTS

- Waxy leaf top with slight fuzziness on underside
- Leaves are basal; flowering stalk emerges in the second year, with leaves alternating up length of stem
- Flowers develop in large, spiny balls that bloom pink to attract pollinators
- Commonly grows in disturbed areas and on the edges of forests in any soil type
- Dried seedpods will latch onto clothes and hair; be careful!
- Roots are best harvested once plant is dying back for winter

RED CLOVER

Trifolium pratense
Family: Fabaceae

Other Names: cowgrass, purple clover

Parts Used: blooms and new leaves

When to Harvest: spring and summer

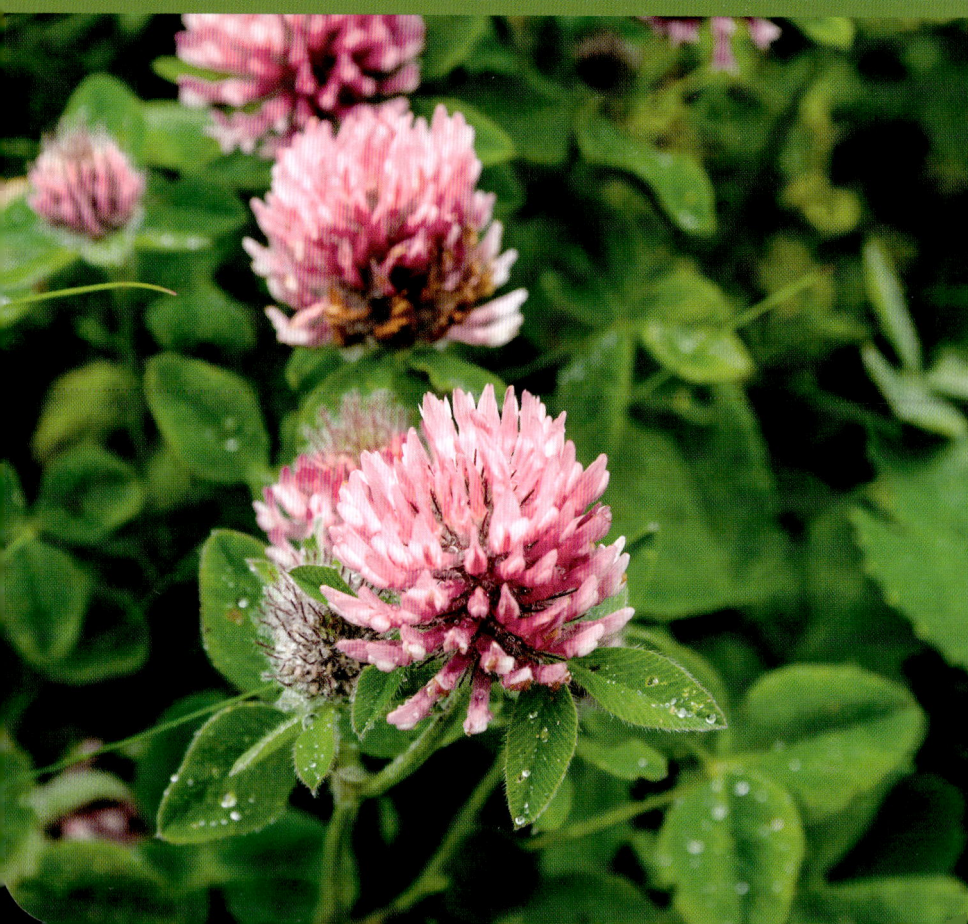

Red clover is a plant I grew up seeing frequently in North Carolina, usually along back roads or in new construction areas. Native to Asia, parts of Africa, and Europe, this plant has naturalized in the Americas, commonly growing in large patches and attracting pollinators in spring and summer. Its pink flowers are often taller and more distinctive than the ubiquitous white clover. Red clover is highly nutritive but has a host of other uses, both internally and externally.

BENEFITS

Nutritive. Rich in vitamins and minerals

Alterative. Restores the normal balance and function of the body's systems and organs

IDENTIFICATION

Red clover is a small herb, growing only about a foot tall, with characteristic pink blooms and clover leaves. As its genus *Trifolium* suggests, red clover's leaves have three ovular leaflets all emerging from the same point. Each leaflet has a unique V-shaped white streak in the middle. Its round flower heads are composed of a cluster of small pink flowers, which dry to a brownish color when the blooms are spent. When compared to white clover, both the flowers and leaves of red clover are much larger and tend to be more erect, especially when in bloom.

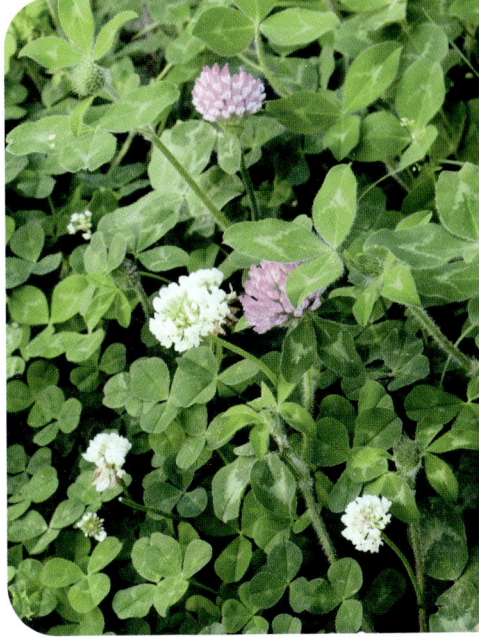

In addition to the difference in color between the blossoms, the leaves of red clover are significantly larger than those of white clover.

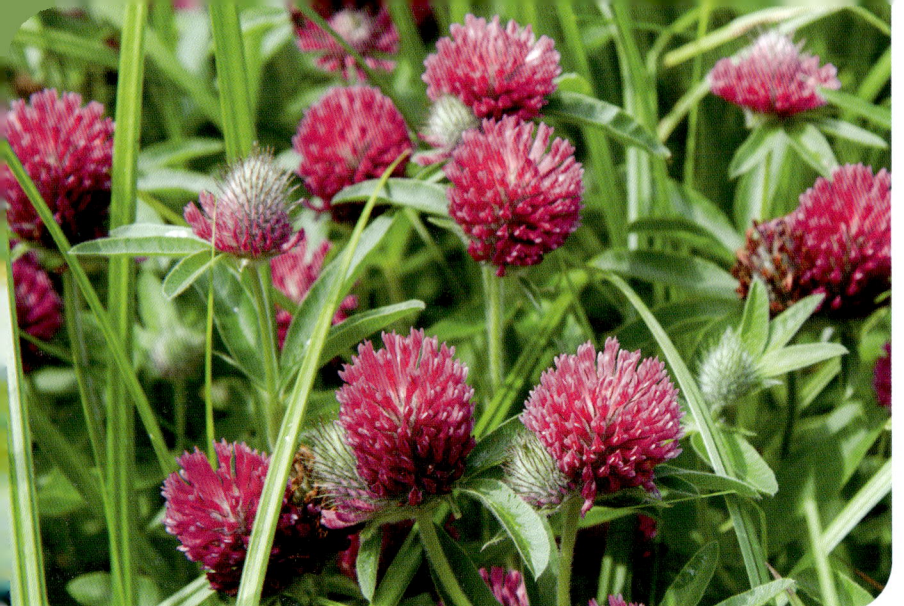

Harvest red clover when the blossoms are fresh and brightly colored.

TRADITIONAL USAGE

Red clover is a moistening, nutritive plant that has often been used alongside other nutrient-dense plants such as oat (*Avena sativa*) to fortify the system and nourish the body. It's rich in trace minerals and B vitamins that can support our organs and bodily processes. The flowers can be boiled into a tea or made into an overnight infusion, which will draw out more nutrients and create a concentrated extract.

As an alterative, red clover moves the blood and the waters of the body. This makes it both a diuretic, increasing urination, and a mild lymphatic, helping stimulate the lymphatic system. With long-term use in a topical oil or salve, alteratives such as red clover are also thought to help ease symptoms of acne, psoriasis, eczema, or a rash.

HARVESTING

Red clover is best harvested when the flowers are bright and pink, before the color has faded. The new leaves are also medicinal, so feel free to cut a few, but prioritize the more potent blooms. Simply pop off the flower heads to harvest; if a plant has many blooms, you can gather the flowers together and cut them as a bundle.

PROCESSING

Red clover dries and stores well. It's best to keep the flower heads intact to slow down oxidization. Some commercial sources for red clover sell crushed, colorless blooms, but you want yours to be vibrant and fresh! Give the blooms a quick rinse and shake before using them, as insects sometimes hitch a ride inside. Use the fresh or dried blooms to make tea or in oils or salves for topical use.

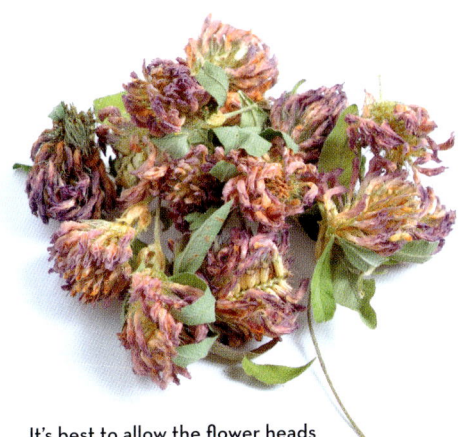

It's best to allow the flower heads to dry intact and then crush them as needed when using.

RED CLOVER FAST FACTS

- Compound leaves formed by three leaflets with a white V-shape on each leaflet
- Bright pink flowers growing in globular clusters
- Grows on roadsides and in meadows, attracting pollinators
- Similar in appearance to white clover, but has different medicinal uses (though both are edible)
- Best harvested in spring and summer
- Leaves can be used, but with less therapeutic effect than flowers

WILD LETTUCE

Lactuca virosa
Family: Asteraceae

Other Names: prickly lettuce, opium lettuce

Parts Used: leaves, stems, and latex

When to Harvest: summer

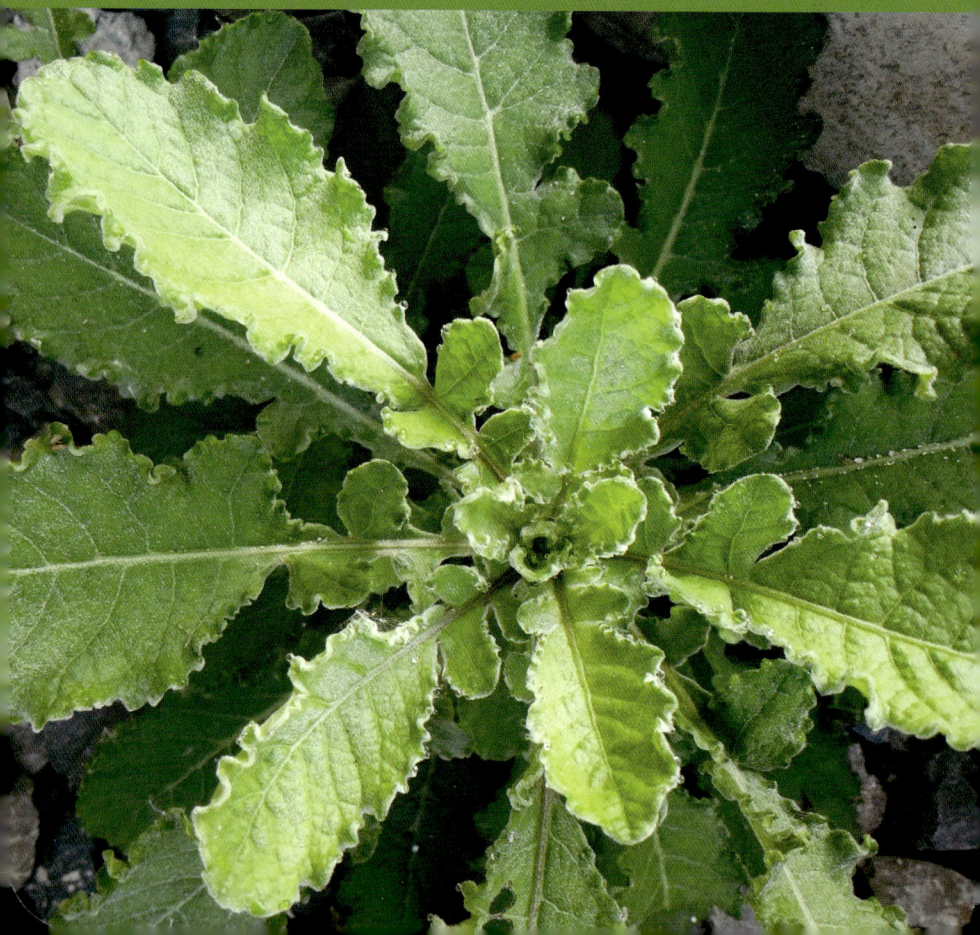

Wild lettuce is a plant I truly considered a weed before learning more about its virtues. Originally native to Europe and parts of India, it now grows across the continental United States and spreads quickly wherever it is introduced. Wild lettuce, like many others members of the Asteraceae family, disperses its fuzzy seed heads in the wind. This unassuming, abundant plant helps soothe and relax the nervous system.

BENEFITS

Analgesic. Pain reliever

Sedative. Promotes calm and sleep

IDENTIFICATION

Wild lettuce is a biennial plant that can grow up to seven feet tall, with yellow flowers in summertime. During its first year of growth, it will grow about a foot tall, with simple, basal leaves emerging from the ground and no flowers. When cut, the leaves and stem release a white latex.

In its second year, a tall flower stalk emerges. The grayish green leaves have a sheathing base, meaning the base of the leaf is wrapped around the stem before growing outward. The leaves have

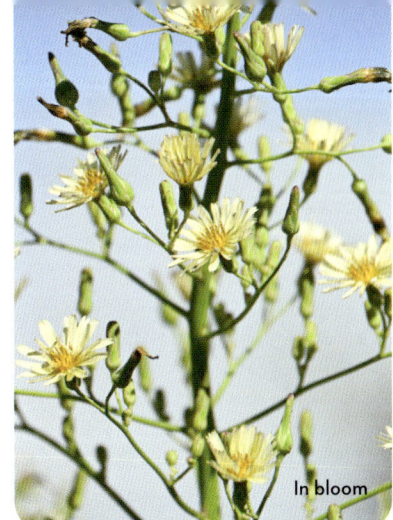

In bloom

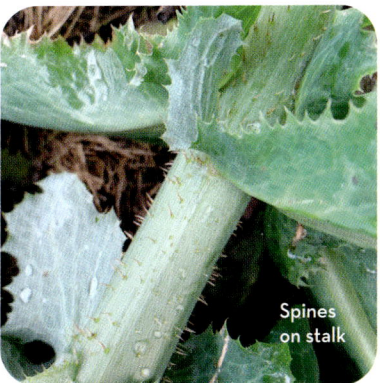

Spines on stalk

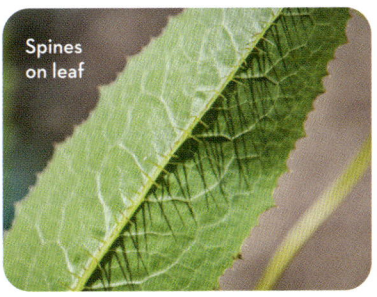

Spines on leaf

jagged, sharp edges and small spines on the central rib running down the middle, which is a helpful identifying feature. The flower buds have small purple spots, and the yellow blooms are purple underneath, as well as on the very ends of the flower petals. The green stem has sharp spines and occasionally has a pattern of red or purple spots.

TRADITIONAL USAGE

Wild lettuce has long been used as a sedative for insomnia, restlessness, and anxiety. The white latex that seeps out from the plant when it's cut contains lactones, which act on the central nervous system to lower activity and relax the nerves. Consuming this plant won't leave you passed out on the floor; rather, it will ease activity in the nervous system, especially for those suffering from the chronic effects of stress. At night, it helps the body relax and alleviates symptoms of insomnia, but in the daytime, it can help ease the tension and anxiety associated with stress and overwork. Wild lettuce's sedative qualities are the result of two compounds: lactucin and lactucopicrin. They have pain-relieving, antispasmodic and calming actions, which can also ease persistent coughs and digestive cramping.

This plant is traditionally used to provide pain relief. Headaches and body pains can be eased by drinking tea or taking concentrated extracts. A fresh-plant tincture is an efficient and easy-to-administer method for both pain relief and nervous system relaxation.

Avoid If Pregnant or Breastfeeding

Use of wild lettuce is not advised during pregnancy or while breastfeeding due to the powerful compounds found in the latex.

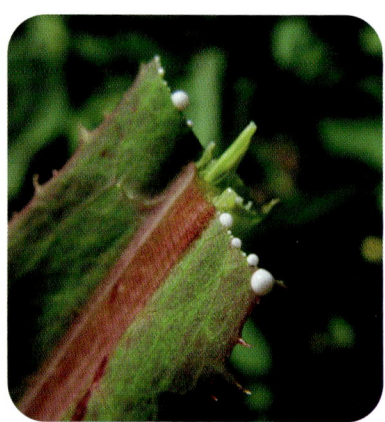

The latex of wild lettuce has potent medicinal qualities and is a helpful identifying feature.

HARVESTING

Wild lettuce is best harvested just before blooming, once the plant has grown a few feet tall in summer. While it can be used after blooming, it's more potent before. Both the leaves and stem contain latex; cut halfway down the plant to harvest both. This will also encourage the plant to branch out, making it easier to harvest later in the season. You can gather this plant in its first year of growth, before it sends up a stem, but I feel it has more energy and impact in the second year.

PROCESSING

I prefer to use wild lettuce fresh. Strip the leaves from the stem and chop up the tender parts of the stem (those that you can easily break). Avoid the older, more fibrous sections of the stem. In a tincture, you can combine both the *menstruum* liquid and plant material in a blender to maximize the surface area and extract all the goodness of the plant. The potent latex will be visible in the finished tincture as a white liquid that settles to the bottom of the jar. If you choose to dry wild lettuce, perhaps to make tea in the future, chop it up well beforehand.

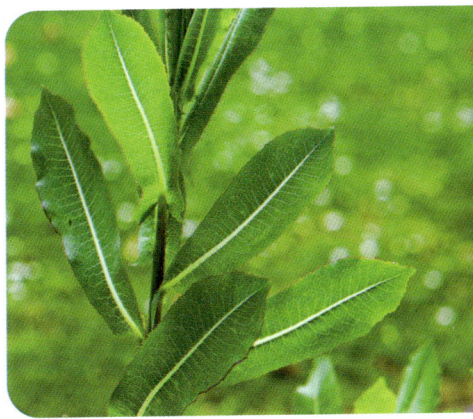

It's best to harvest wild lettuce in its second year, when it produces a flowering stalk.

WILD LETTUCE FAST FACTS

- Center rib of leaf has a line of spines, as do the leaf edges
- Biennial; plant grows up to seven feet tall in second year
- Blooms are clusters of yellow flowers that ripen to fluffy seed heads and blow away in wind
- Green stem, sometimes blotched with red and purple spots; spines along stem
- When cut, all parts exude white latex
- Commonly growing in fields and disturbed areas

SPANISH NEEDLE

Bidens alba, Bidens pilosa, Bidens frondosa
Family: Asteraceae

Other Names: margarita, bidens, beggarsticks, romerillo

Parts Used: new leaf growth and flowers

When to Harvest: spring, summer, and fall

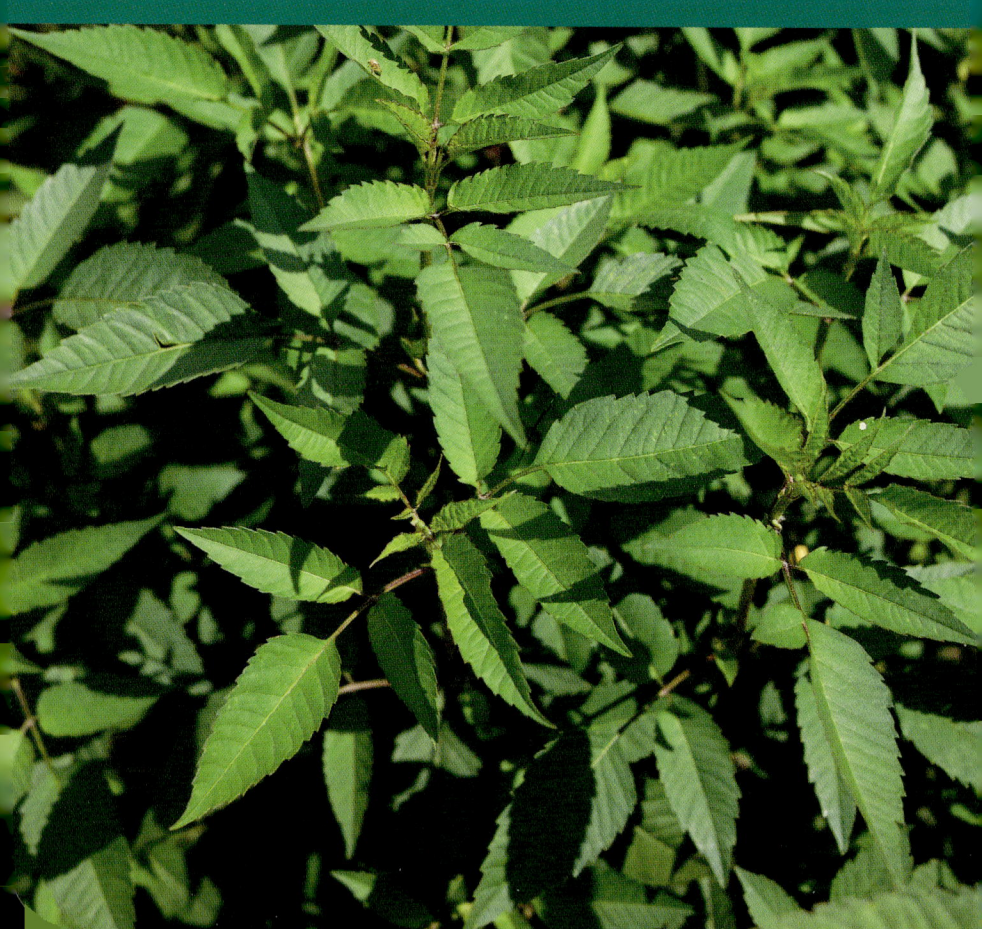

Spanish needle goes by many names. I learned one of its Spanish names, *margarita*, from my grandparents and elders in Puerto Rico. From herbalists in North Carolina, I came to know it as *bidens*. Here we'll refer to it as Spanish needle, a common English name and one that's popular in parts of the Caribbean as well. Spanish needle is both a food and a medicine, but it can also be aggressively invasive. Some states even prohibit the sale of the seeds to prevent continued spread, so use the species native to whatever area you're in. I've worked mostly with *Bidens alba*, *B. pilosa*, and *B. frondosa* (this species is often referred to by names other than Spanish needle, but it can be used interchangeably).

BENEFITS

Nutritive. Rich in vitamins and minerals

Antibiotic. Kills bacteria or inhibits their growth

Diuretic. Helps the body eliminate excess water through increased urination

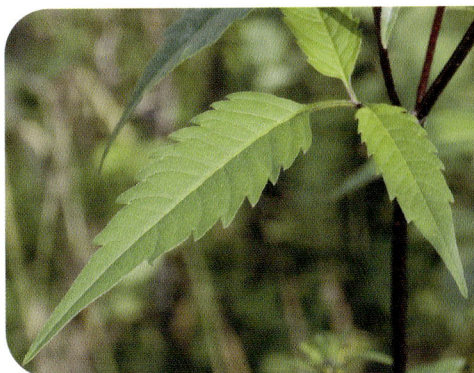

Gather the leaves to use for medicine or as a tasy potherb before the plant has begun to bloom.

IDENTIFICATION

Though there are many species of bidens, I'll focus on *Bidens frondosa*, a species that grows throughout North America. While there is some overlap with other species, each is botanically unique. Spanish needle is in the Asteraceae family and has an odd number of compound, pinnate leaves. The leaves are a rich green color and serrated. The stem of the plant tends to have a dark purplish hue that continues into the petiole as well. It can grow anywhere from two to six feet tall in a single season.

Spanish needle produces orange flower heads with yellow petals. There can be multiple blooms, generally smaller than an inch in size, growing from several points on the same plant. After blooming, the seedpods develop in clusters. The pods are rectangular and brownish black with two small "horns" on one side. This allows the seeds to latch onto clothes, hair, and skin, helping the plant distribute itself. As the plant gets older, it will develop more purple spots along the leaves, before eventually dying back in winter.

Be aware of where you harvest this plant, as it can pull chemicals and toxins from the soil. It can grow in concrete and in polluted areas like roadsides, but also grows near trails and drainage areas. While it's tolerant of dryness, it is commonly found in moist soils.

TRADITIONAL USAGE

One of the primary uses of Spanish needle is as a nutritive herb. The leaves are rich in protein, zinc, iron, and various trace minerals that fortify and nourish the body. It can be eaten raw or lightly cooked and added to dishes as a potherb with a very mild flavor. Spanish needle is commonly included in dishes served postpartum to help nourish and heal the body after the intense process of childbirth. It's also beneficial for people with anemia or general low energy, and individuals who are recovering from medical procedures or accidents.

Spanish needle has antibiotic qualities and an affinity for smooth muscle tissue, which makes it a powerful ally for easing infections in the gums, stomach, urinary tract, and colon. The leaves can be chewed and held in the mouth to help address gum infections, toothache, and oral cuts. Making a tea or tincturing can extract these properties as well. It's also astringent and tonifying, helping recovery from diarrhea and extensive digestive upset.

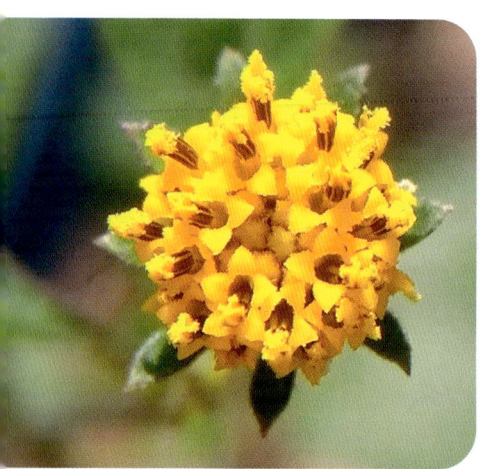

The blooms of Spanish needle can be used in much the same way as the leaves.

In the Caribbean, this plant is combined with many others to create a rich decoction popularly known as a root tonic, which is used to address everything from general pain and low energy to low immune function and fever. The flowers can be boiled as a general wellness tonic to regulate kidney, digestive, and liver function.

HARVESTING

Harvesting this plant helps maintain a stable population and prevents it from going to seed excessively. The leaves are best gathered before the plant blooms. Tender green shoots can be clipped with pruners or even plucked off with your hands, a sign the plant growth is not yet overly fibrous and tough. Harvest blooms in the same way, simply by popping them off the stem. Spanish needle petals will fall off soon after they bloom, but the flower buds dry well or can be used fresh to brew tea or make tinctures.

Spanish needle can be harvested throughout the year; in temperate climates it will start going to seed in late summer but will continue providing harvests until frost hits. If you pull up the entire plant to limit its growth in the area, discard the roots and select good quality, green leaves from the stem, especially the tender shoots.

PREPARATION

Spanish needle is an excellent edible green, and I especially love to add it to soups. As a nutritive, it's great to include in vinegars and pesto. I've even had luck drying and powdering the leaves and sprinkling them into different dishes. For the most potent preparation, a simple decoction will extract the medicinal compounds from this plant efficiently and yield a rich green herbal flavor. For tincture making, it's best to use fresh Spanish needle. When processing, discard overly fibrous stems and focus on the flowers, leaves, and tender shoots.

SPANISH NEEDLE FAST FACTS

- Leaves are compound, pinnate
- Found in disturbed areas such as roadsides, trails, and construction sites
- Purple petiole and stem
- Orange flower heads with yellow petals and dry, brown seed clusters that latch onto clothing easily
- Plant can grow anywhere from two feet to six feet tall
- Great as both food and medicine, edible raw and cooked

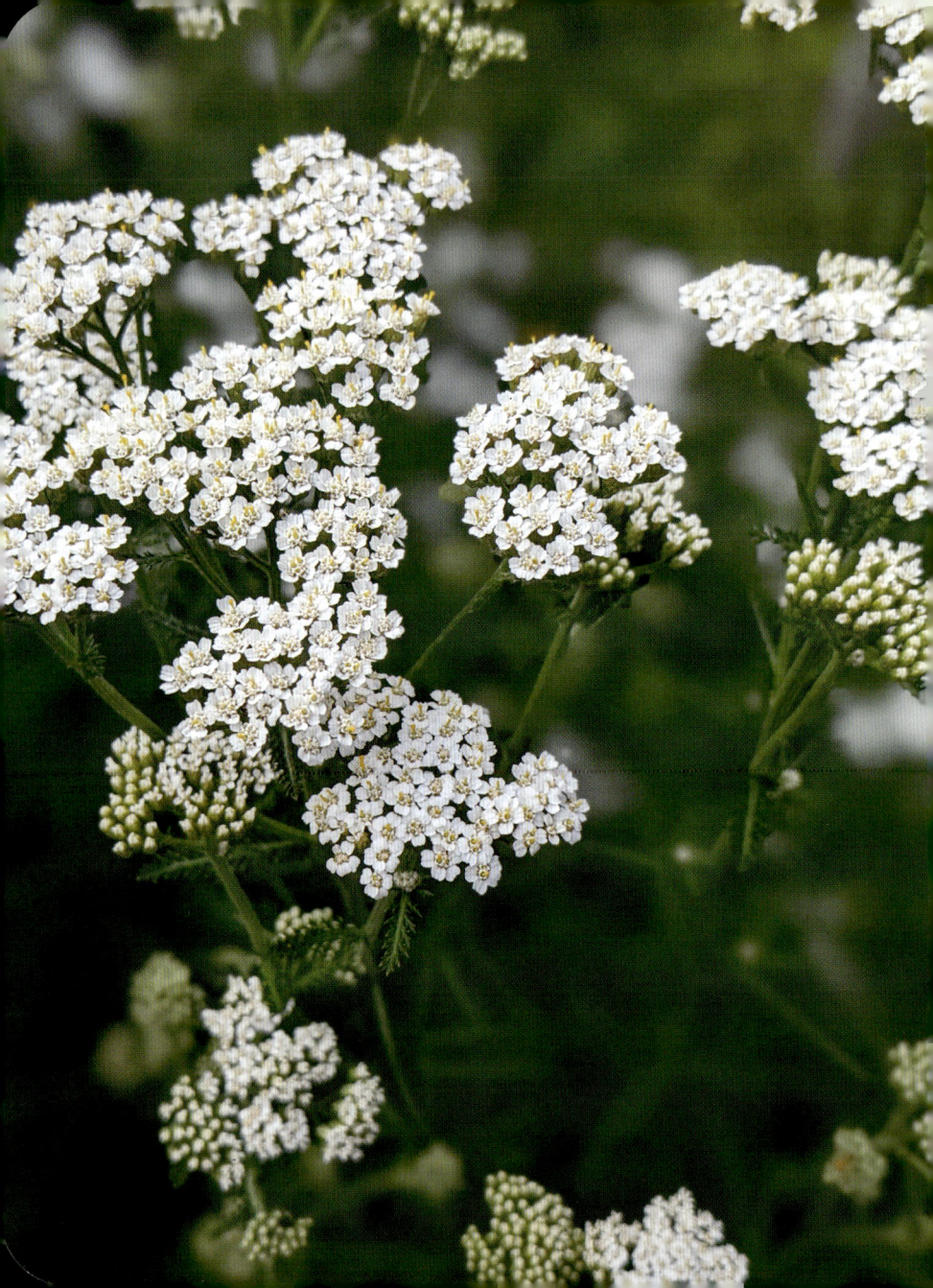

YARROW

Achillea millefolium
Family: Asteraceae

Other Names: soldierwort, woundwort

Parts Used: flower heads and occasionally leaves

When to Use: summer

Yarrow was among the first plants I grew in my garden. An easy-to-grow perennial, the tiny plant I put in the ground ended up about three feet wide, developing into a patch that was covered in blooms throughout the summer months. Native to the Americas and throughout Asia and Europe, yarrow is a favorite for butterflies and other pollinators, and soon my yard was abuzz with insect life. But it's much more than a nice garden perennial—yarrow is a soothing and aromatic medicine that can be used both externally and internally.

BENEFITS

Styptic. Stops bleeding

Diaphoretic. Increases sweating to break fever

Bitter. Stimulates digestion and acts on the liver

Vulnerary. Stimulates wound healing when used topically

IDENTIFICATION

Yarrow's leaves are fernlike, with many tiny leaflets. This feature earned yarrow the species name *millefolium* or "thousand leaves." Its delicate leaves emerge directly from the soil, not developing a central stem until the flowering stalk emerges and the leaves begin to grow alternately up the stem. Yarrow blooms in white clusters composed of many tiny

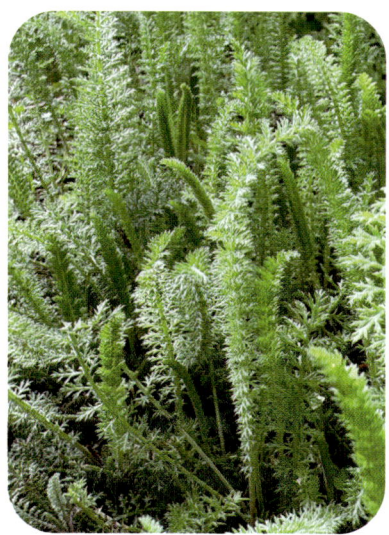

The fernlike leaves of yarrow grow directly from the ground without a central stem.

flowers; the flat-headed flower clusters, called corymbs, consist of branching stems grouped together to make an even, rounded surface of blooms. When the white flowers dry out, they turn brown and remain on the flower stalk through winter. Though the seeds will germinate, this plant also spreads through rhizome growth underground. When crushed, both the leaves and flowers emit a menthol-like aroma. Yarrow likes to grow in meadows and forest edges and sometimes grows near low-traffic roadsides.

TRADITIONAL USAGE

Yarrow is used in many ways, but the most unique is as a topical medicine. Historically, the fresh blooms have been crushed and applied to open wounds to stop bleeding on battlefields, earning it the name *soldierwort* in some places. It's a powerful styptic, meaning it stops bleeding by encouraging the coagulation of blood. In less dire situations it's great for small cuts and scrapes. It's also a vulnerary and can be made into oils and salves to help stimulate wound healing. The combination of aromatic oils and alkaloids found in yarrow help facilitate the healing process.

Internally, yarrow is used as a diaphoretic to induce sweating and break a fever, most commonly in the form of a tea. For more acute cases, use yarrow as a tincture in combination with other herbs.

As an aromatic bitter, yarrow can also be taken to stimulate saliva production and aid the digestive system. A little yarrow tea or tincture before or after a meal can be helpful for people with sluggish digestion or who experience indigestion after eating.

HARVESTING

Keep an eye on the yarrow plant as the flowers begin to emerge in summer, and harvest when the buds first open. Choose fresh flowers; make sure none of them are browning before you harvest, as you want new blooms. The leaves can be harvested regardless of whether the plant is blooming, though I generally prefer to work with the flowers. Cut the entire stem at the base. If you leave the stem attached it will eventually decompose on the plant, draining the plant's energy in the process. Cutting the full stem also makes it easier to hang to dry; simply tie a string around the long stems.

PROCESSING

To use in salves and oil, dry the flowers first, as the water content of fresh plants can lead to spoilage. Before drying, wash the flowers thoroughly and pull apart the clusters a bit to allow the air to circulate as they dry. You can make a tincture using fresh or dried flowers; simply crush up the flowers well before tincturing.

To use the leaves, crush them and make a simple infusion. The dried leaves can also be infused into oil as you would with the flowers or you can crush the fresh leaves and use them as a topical poultice.

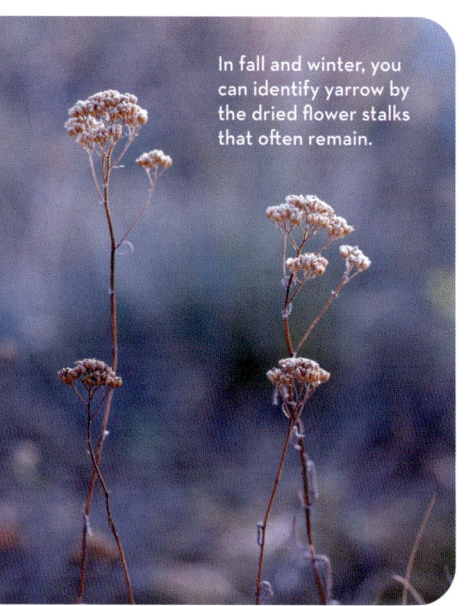

In fall and winter, you can identify yarrow by the dried flower stalks that often remain.

YARROW FAST FACTS

- White flowers growing in a flat, slightly rounded cluster
- Fine, fernlike leaves emerging directly from soil
- Leaves alternate up stem when blooming in summer and fall
- Common along forest edges and meadows
- Best harvested in summer when first blooms emerge
- Make sure to leave some flower heads for pollinators!

MOTHERWORT

Leonurus cardiaca
Family: Lamiaceae

Other Names: throw wort, lion's tail

Parts Used: leaves and flowering aerial parts

When to Harvest: summer

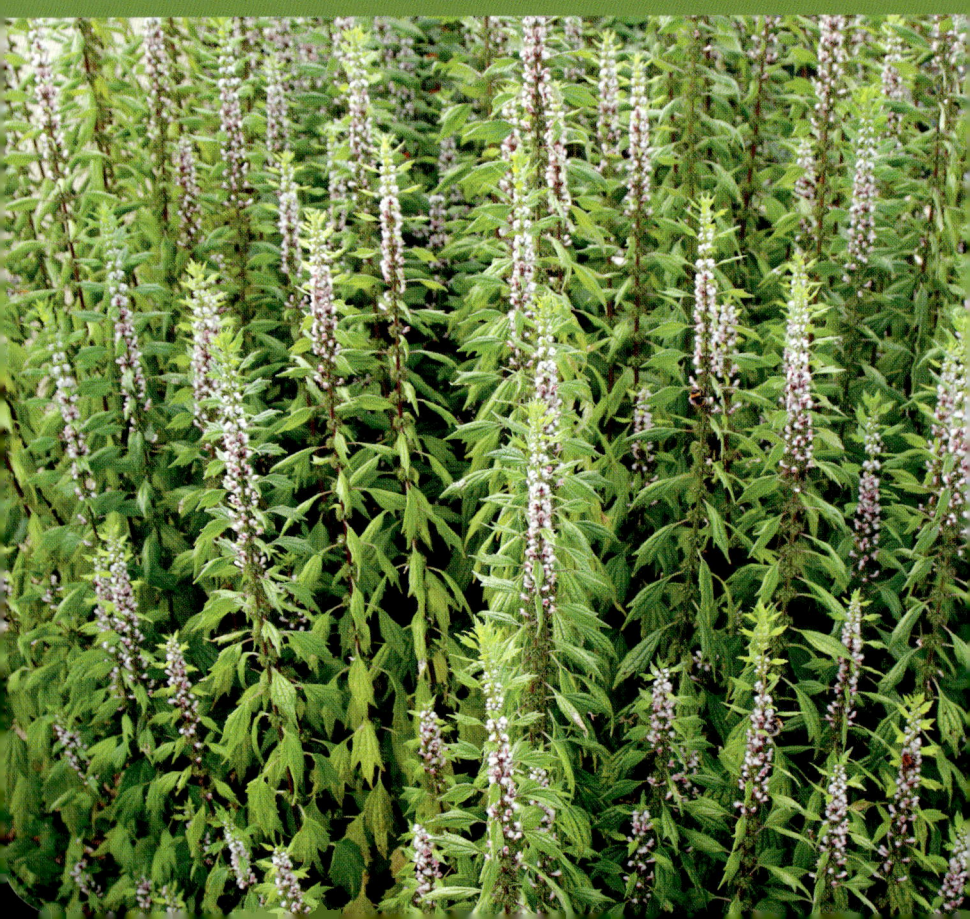

Motherwort is a powerful ally for mothers, folks with heartache, and truly anyone with a frazzled nervous system. It's commonly planted in gardens or found growing wild and naturalized in disturbed areas across North America. Its ability to self-sow ensures that it can be harvested year after year. The pollinators love it, too, flocking to its bright pink flowers on a sunny day. Native to Europe and Asia, motherwort has long been used as a tonic herb that remedies issues of the nervous and reproductive systems. It has become one of my favorites and is a great medicinal support for anyone stressed, overworked, and in need of deeper rest and heart medicine.

BENEFITS

Cardiovascular tonic. Supports the cardiovascular system

Nervine. Supports the nervous system

Emmenagogue. Stimulates or increases menstruation

Hypotensive. Lowers blood pressure

Diaphoretic. Increases sweating to break fever

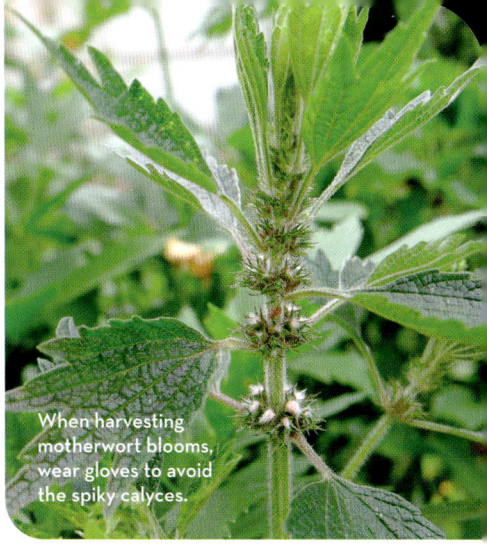

When harvesting motherwort blooms, wear gloves to avoid the spiky calyces.

IDENTIFICATION

Motherwort plants can grow up to four feet tall. The leaves are light green, and when blooming its flowers are pink. The leaves are opposite like many other mint family plants. They are shallowly lobed and look similar to mugwort but are a bit wider and distinctly fuzzier. Younger leaves have a slightly more angular shape. Both the leaves and the square stem are covered in a soft, fine hair. The blooming flowers that emerge on the upper part of the plant are surrounded by spiky calyces, a helpful identifying feature and something to keep in mind when harvesting. This plant blooms through summer and likes to grow in disturbed areas, in gardens, or anywhere it has been previously planted, as it self-seeds.

Avoid If Pregnant or Taking Heart Medication

Motherwort should not be taken while pregnant or if you're trying to become pregnant. It can also interact with some heart medications, so be sure to consult with a healthcare provider before consuming.

TRADITIONAL USAGE

Motherwort has traditionally been used by mothers suffering from stress, anxiety, and restlessness. Do you know who else is stressed, restless, and occasionally suffering from anxiety? Almost everyone! While its name might make you think it is only for mothers or women, this is a plant for folks with any type of body. It's the perfect nourishing and calming remedy during times of stress and a favorite of mine for general nervous system wellness. It's an excellent daily tonic; it doesn't cause drowsiness, but nourishes and protects the nervous system from the long-term effects of stress. It's especially powerful for the heart, in both a physical and a spiritual sense. I include it in formulas for grief and emotional exhaustion alongside other heart tonics, such as mimosa (page 177). Its flavor is mild and tends to blend well with others, but it can make a nice vegetable glycerin extract by itself.

This plant is also a hypotensive, meaning it helps lower blood pressure. It's ideal for folks dealing with everyday stressors that elevate their blood pressure and can help support those dealing with consistently high blood pressure and heart issues. However, motherwort can interfere with some heart medications, so always check with a healthcare expert to ensure it's a safe option for you. It doesn't interact with many medications, but its profound effect on the heart means it's best to be mindful.

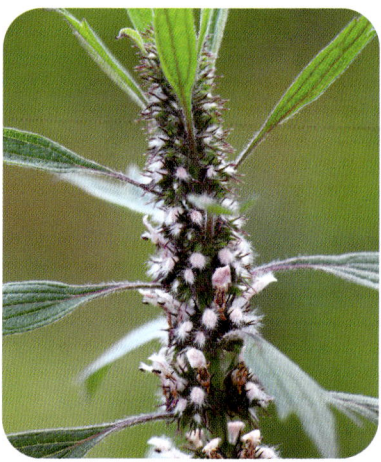

Motherwort blossoms have a mild flavor that pairs well with glycerin preparations.

Motherwort has an affinity for the uterus and has often been made into a tea used to stimulate menses and ease the smooth muscle cramping caused by menstrual cycles. Contrary to what the name might lead you to believe, it should generally be avoided by pregnant people because of these stimulant properties. It is strengthening as a tonic for the uterus, helping alleviate some symptoms of premenstrual syndrome.

HARVESTING

Gather motherwort in summer when it flowers, cutting about half a foot down from the top of the plant just above a leaf node. This stimulates more growth and encourages another harvest later in the season. Be aware of the spiky calyces and wear gloves! Avoid leaves lower on the plant, focusing on the newer growth toward the top. The same applies to the stems—the older growth is more fibrous and less potent.

PREPARATION

Motherwort flowers and leaves are excellent prepared as a tea and a tincture. A simple tincture in alcohol works, or use vegetable glycerin if you prefer a sweeter flavor. A tincture can be made from fresh or dried herb, and its mild flavor is easy to add to blends or drinks. I use motherwort frequently in my practice because heart and nervous system support are vital. Motherwort tea and a little honey is never a bad idea!

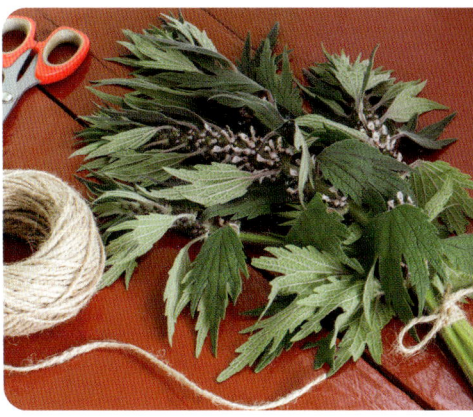

Motherwort blossoms dry well for future use. Tie the cut stalks together with twine and hang in a warm, dry place with good airflow.

MOTHERWORT FAST FACTS

- Square stem with opposite leaves
- Leaves vary with age: sharp, angled lobes at new growth, becoming rounder at old growth
- Leaves are soft and fuzzy
- Pink flowers emerge from spiky calyces around leaf nodes
- Plant can grow up to six feet tall
- Common in disturbed areas, escaped from gardens, and forest edges

HORSETAIL

Equisetum spp.
Family: Equisetaceae

Other Names: shavegrass

Parts Used: all aerial parts

When to Harvest: spring through summer

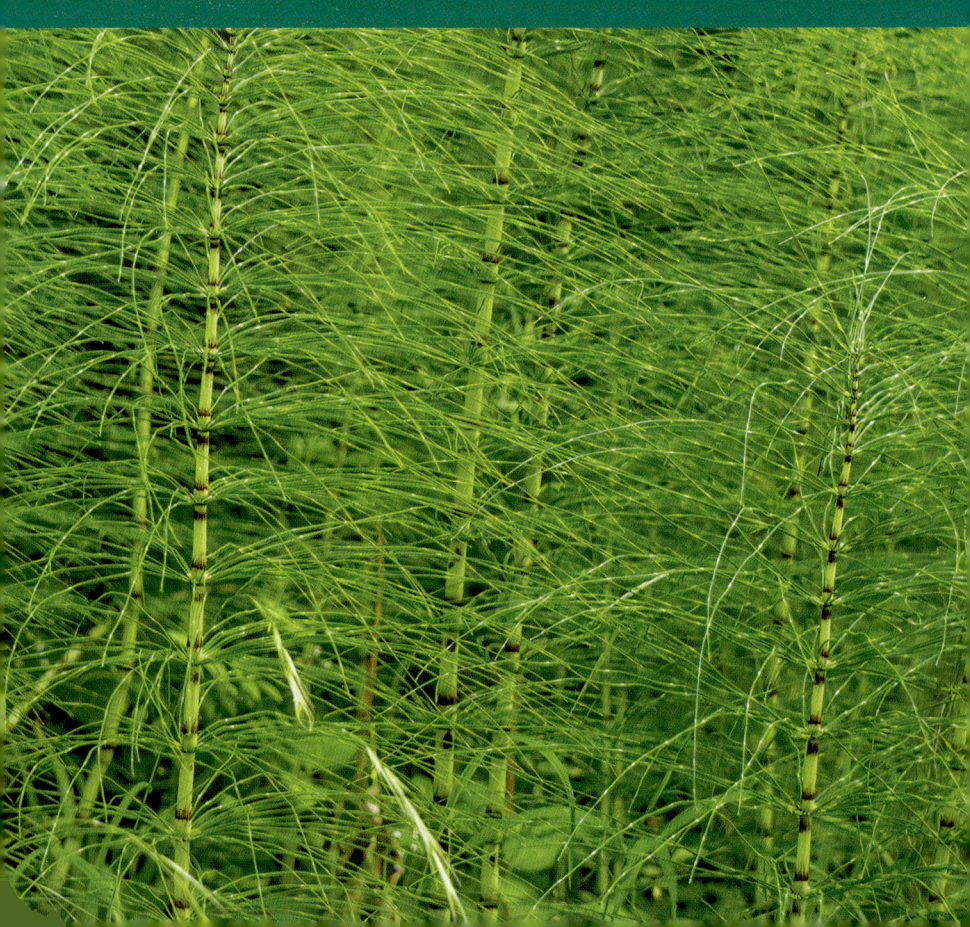

At first glance, this fascinating plant looks like a tiny bamboo shoot or even a fern. Horsetail is in the Equisetaceae family, the last descendant of the Equisetales, a prehistoric plant family dating back to 375 million years ago. Though they used to grow almost 100 feet tall, horsetails now average 2 to 3 feet, although some species, such as *Equisetum giganteum*, reach up to 10 feet. When I come across horsetail in the wild, I like to imagine the time when they would have towered over me. This plant is a beautiful reminder of the land's ancient past and a good source of medicine.

BENEFITS

Nutritive. Rich in vitamins and minerals

Diuretic. Helps the body eliminate excess water through increased urination

Musculoskeletal tonic. Supports the bones, muscles, and joints

IDENTIFICATION

Horsetail has two stages of growth through the year. In spring, a light brown stem emerges with a conelike flowering head at the tip. This "flower" emits spores, which are one way this plant reproduces. This stem eventually dies back, and stiff, green vegetative growth will emerge. The "leaves" appear as brown sheaths around the joints of the plant, every few inches along the stem. The stem is green with vertical ridges that are very rough when crushed or scratched. Horsetails can grow bare as a single shoot or can display whorled leaf structures, similar in appearance to pine needles, that grow up the stem. The plant is hollow, which differentiates it from possible look-alikes such as rushes

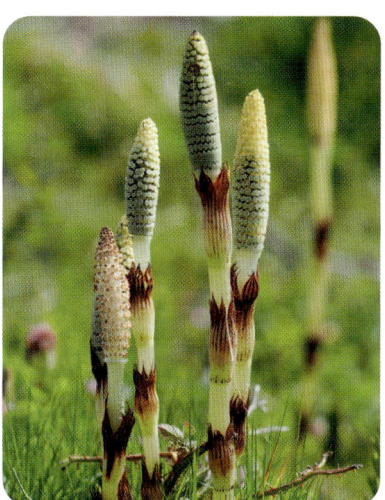

Horsetail's spore-producing flowering heads emerge in spring but aren't good sources of medicine.

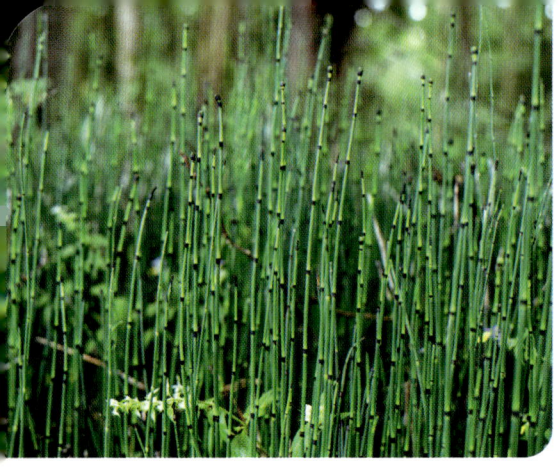
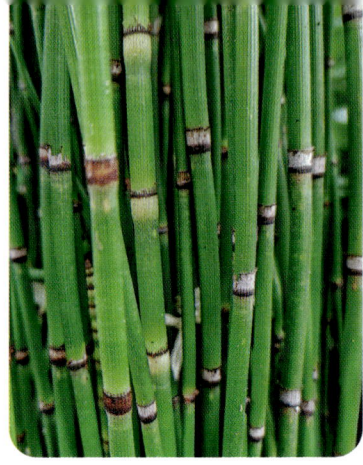

Horsetail can grow as a single shoot (above) or produce needlelike leaf structures.

If you bend horsetail at a node, you'll notice that it's surprisingly flexible.

that you may find in similar environments. Horsetail likes to grow in moist areas where water gathers but can also grow in dry, rocky soils throughout temperate North America.

TRADITIONAL USAGE

Horsetail is a great example of the *doctrine of signatures*, which suggests that the physical traits of plants relate to their medicinal usage. For instance, walnuts, which are good for brain health, are shaped like tiny brains. When boiled, chaney root (*Smilax balbisiana*) releases a blood red color, which is fitting because it is traditionally used to nourish the blood. When horsetail is bent, it's surprisingly supple. If you bend it at the joint, it has the same flexible quality as connective tissue. And sure enough, this plant is used to support bone and connective tissue health, nourishing the entire musculoskeletal system. Horsetail is rich in calcium and silica, both of which are vital to joint and bone health—and also nourish the skin, hair, and nails.

Horsetail is traditionally boiled and made into tea but can be tinctured in alcohol. When tinctured, it acts as a diuretic, encouraging urination and releasing excess water from the body. It is nourishing to the kidneys and even aids the connective tissue of the bladder. Externally, horsetail's mineral content can be used to strengthen the hair and nails by being made into a wash—essentially a tea poured over the hair that nourishes your fingernails and skin in the process (see page 235).

HARVESTING

The spore-spreading part of the plant that first emerges from the ground isn't ideal for medicine; it's best to harvest the green, vegetative part that marks the second stage of its lifecycle. You can harvest horsetail from the ground, pulling it up from the root because it grows in such abundance. However, it will probably be back in short order, as the plant can repropagate itself from tiny pieces of rhizome.

PROCESSING

Horsetail dries very easily with good airflow and warmth. The plant is very fibrous, so before use it's best to break it into smaller pieces, either by pulling at the sheath located at each node or by using scissors. When you purchase horsetail commercially, it is often processed into tiny pieces, but I prefer to leave it in large chunks, breaking them down further just before using. If tincturing, add a little water, even if the plant is fresh, because it's not very high in water content.

HORSETAIL FAST FACTS

- Commonly grows in wet places; it pulls up silica and potentially other chemicals as well; be mindful of where you're harvesting from and, if near water, what is upstream
- Some (but not all) plants have whorled needlelike spokes growing around shoot
- Shoots have "leaves" that appear as gray or black sheaths every few inches up plant
- Shoots are hollow and flexible when bent at joints
- In spring, look for brown shoot with a conical shape atop it; this spore-releasing part of plant doesn't have much medicinal value
- Bamboolike growth directly from ground, ranging from one to six feet depending on species

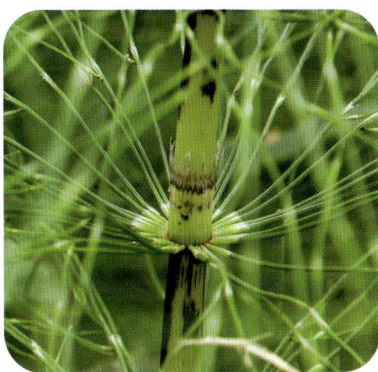

Horsetail "leaves" grow as sheaths around the joint of the plant.

WILD ROSE

Rosa spp.
Family: Rosaceae

Other Names: rose, beach rose

Parts Used: leaves, petals, and fruits

When to Harvest: summer and fall

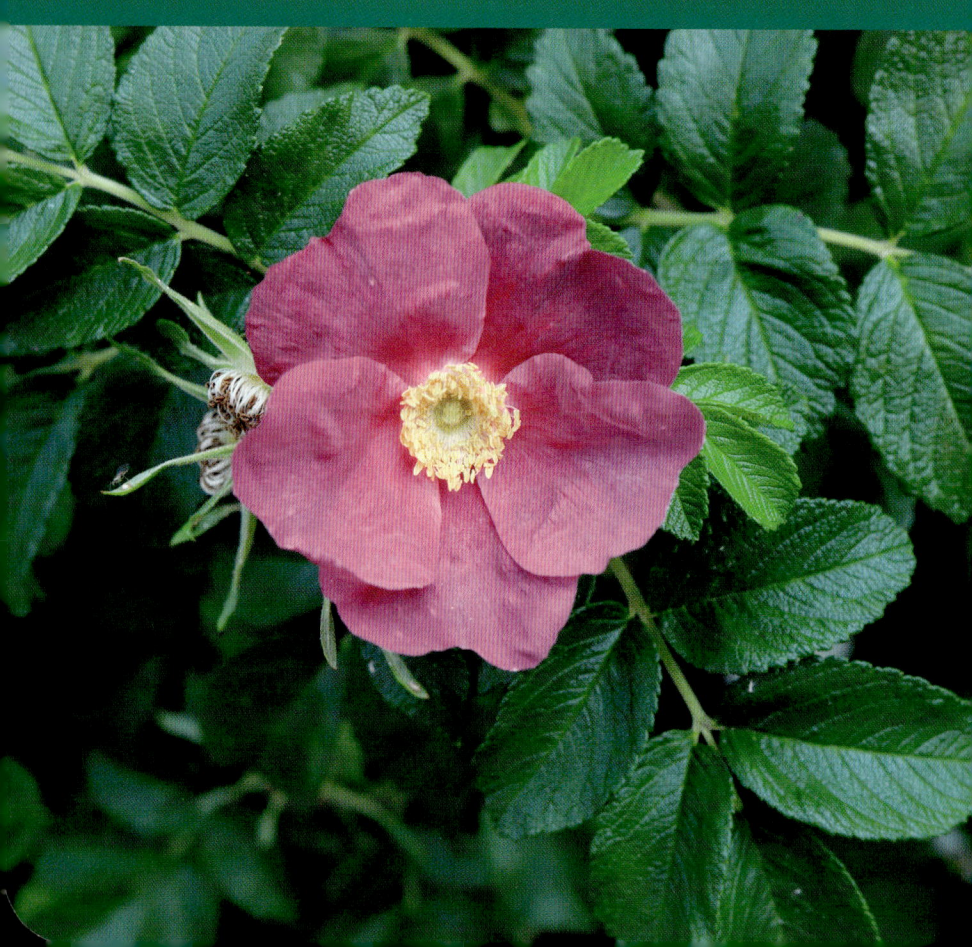

In addition to being a symbol for love and a beloved garden staple, roses have powerful medicinal qualities. The aromatic petals and sour, bright fruits are the most commonly used parts of the plant, but the intricately textured leaves can also be used for healing purposes. The petals contain geraniol, which gives them their signature aroma and provides great medicinal value as well.

Rose is a good example of an aromatic medicine that has effects beyond the physical. When we inhale a scent, the brain's *limbic system* is activated. This part of the brain is responsible for regulating emotions, memory, and other functions. Our emotional, spiritual, and physical health are all interconnected, and rose is a plant that can affect the many realms within ourselves.

BENEFITS

Anxiolytic. Eases anxiety

Mild astringent. Tonifies skin and smooth muscle tissue

Nutritive. Rich in vitamins and minerals

IDENTIFICATION

Rosebushes tend to grow between three and four feet tall. Wild species may be smaller, growing just one foot tall. Most species have flowers with five petals. Wild species are always pink, while ornamental varieties can be any of a rainbow of different colors, including white and yellow. Rose leaves are arranged in opposite pairs of leaflets, generally two or three pairs, with a single leaf at the top. The leaves are serrated. Some species, such as *Rosa rugosa*, have distinct and deeply textured leaves, while others are smoother. One of the easiest identifiers of a rose

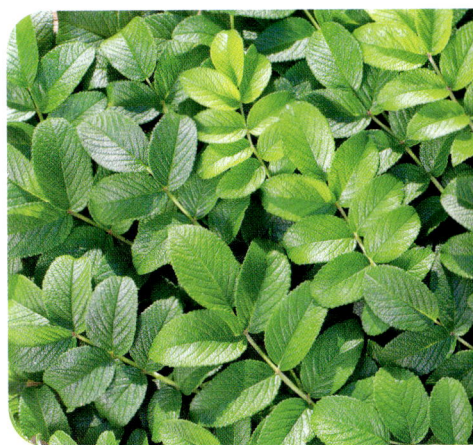

Rose leaves are compound and can be deeply textured, depending on the species.

is the thorns running up the stem. You will see both large, firm spikes and smaller, fine hairs that are just as prickly. The leaves may also have a few spikes underneath. The calyx surrounding the petals before blooming and the flower stems are both covered in spikes as well. For a plant associated with love, it's very prickly!

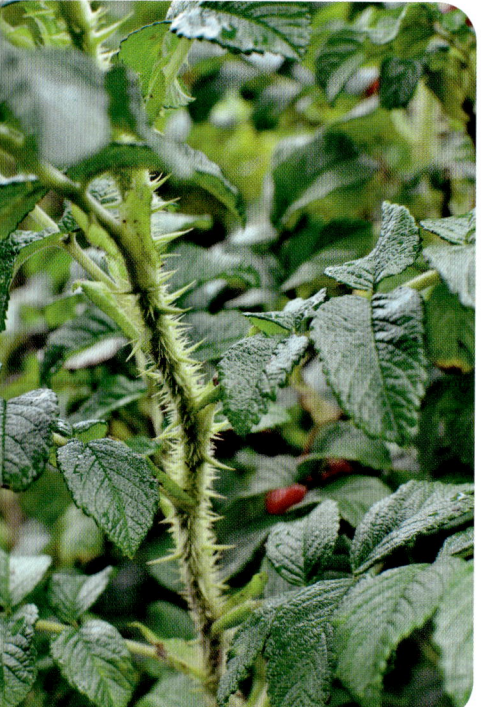

Roses are famous for their thorns, so harvest with care.

TRADITIONAL USAGE

Rose petals are traditionally made into a tea for calming purposes. Rose petal tea is one of my favorites for soothing the nervous system, easing into relaxation after a long day of work and right before bed. The medicinal actions of rose petals are mild, but the aromatic qualities help relax the muscles and ease stress. Like the rest of the plant, rose petals are cooling, soothing, and mildly drying; they can help ease an upset stomach and heat-related ailments. If you're feeling dehydrated after a long day outside, some refreshing rose petal tea can help.

Rose petals are the perfect complementary herb, augmenting and supporting other herbs that have stronger medicinal qualities. Try rose with motherwort (page 122) for anxiety, with mimosa (page 177) as an uplifting brew for emotional distress, or with linden (page 190) for sleep- and restlessness.

Rose petals and leaves are also astringent, helping tonify and tighten tissue. For example, sinus tissue might be overly relaxed due to allergies, but astringent medicine can help contract it, easing a runny nose or scratchy throat. Rose leaves are more astringent than the petals, and they can be boiled and drunk for this purpose. In spring, the new leaf shoots can be a regulating tonic for the stomach after a cold winter, and are traditionally eaten by Indigenous peoples in North America.

The fruits (rose hips) are high in vitamin C and antioxidants and are traditionally boiled into a remedy for colds and flu in winter. Boil the ripe red fruits and mix them with honey to make a delicious sweet-and-sour syrup that can be used for sore throat and general winter wellness. Rose hips are filled with seeds and small hairs that can potentially be irritating, so be sure to strain the liquid well.

HARVESTING

Roses are frequently used for landscaping and are often seen outside of commercial spaces, in front of houses, in recreational areas, and at beaches. There are over a hundred different species of rose, and thousands of different varieties have been bred for showy petals, color variation, compact shrub growth, and many other traits. You can use any species of rose medicinally, but make sure you know whether the plant has been treated with pesticides or other chemicals. As a common landscaping plant, it's frequently treated with chemicals in public and residential spaces, so you want to be completely certain about your source.

Roses generally bloom in early summer through fall, depending on your area. Harvest rose petals as they begin to open, within a day or two of the flowers unfurling, as this is when their aroma is strongest. You can harvest the

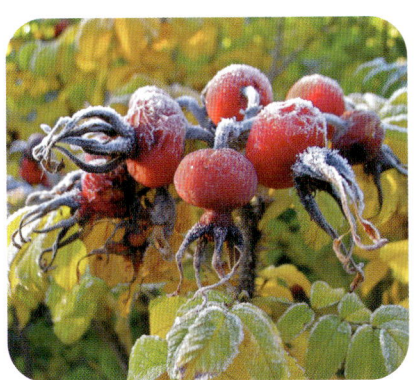

Rose hips are often sweeter after the first frost.

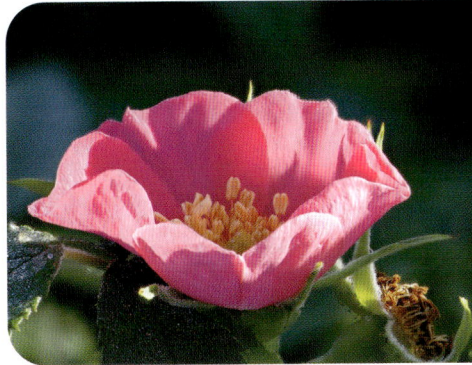

Gather rose blossoms shortly after they open, when they're at their most aromatic.

entire flower head along with the calyx underneath. Leave some flowers behind for pollinators, though. Remember that later in the season they'll ripen into tangy rose hips! Gather rose hips after the first frost, which helps convert the tannins into sugars and creates a sweeter fruit. Fresh leaf shoots come up in spring; if you wish to use them as a potherb, harvest when they are tender and easy to pop off the plant.

WILD ROSE FAST FACTS

- Pinnate leaves with an odd number of leaflets (pairs of opposite leaflets with a single leaflet at the end)
- Some varieties are very low-growing, almost like a ground cover, while others grow tall like shrubs
- Both thorns and small hairs along stem and bottoms of leaves
- Blooms and fruits are the primary medicinal parts
- All species of rose are edible and medicinal
- Blooms can be harvested year-round whenever first unfurling; fruits best after first frost

PREPARATION

Dried rose petals are a bit more potent than the fresh, water-dense petals. The petals dry easily, while rose hips take a bit longer to dry fully. Make a cut into the fruit to allow them to dry faster. Rose petal tea is an easy preparation that captures the beautiful aroma of the petals. Rose hips need to be decocted to release their compounds. A nice rolling boil for 5 to 10 minutes will extract that tangy, vitamin C–rich flavor. I love boiling rose hips into a concentrated decoction and then mixing it with rose honey to make an immersive rose experience. Sweet and aromatic! Rose petals can be added to any dishes you like; powder them or add them fresh or dried to your favorite recipes.

ELDERBERRY

Sambucus canadensis, Sambucus nigra, Sambucus mexicana
Family: Adoxaceae

Other Names: elder, sauco

Parts Used: ripe berries, flowers, and leaves

When to Harvest: spring and summer

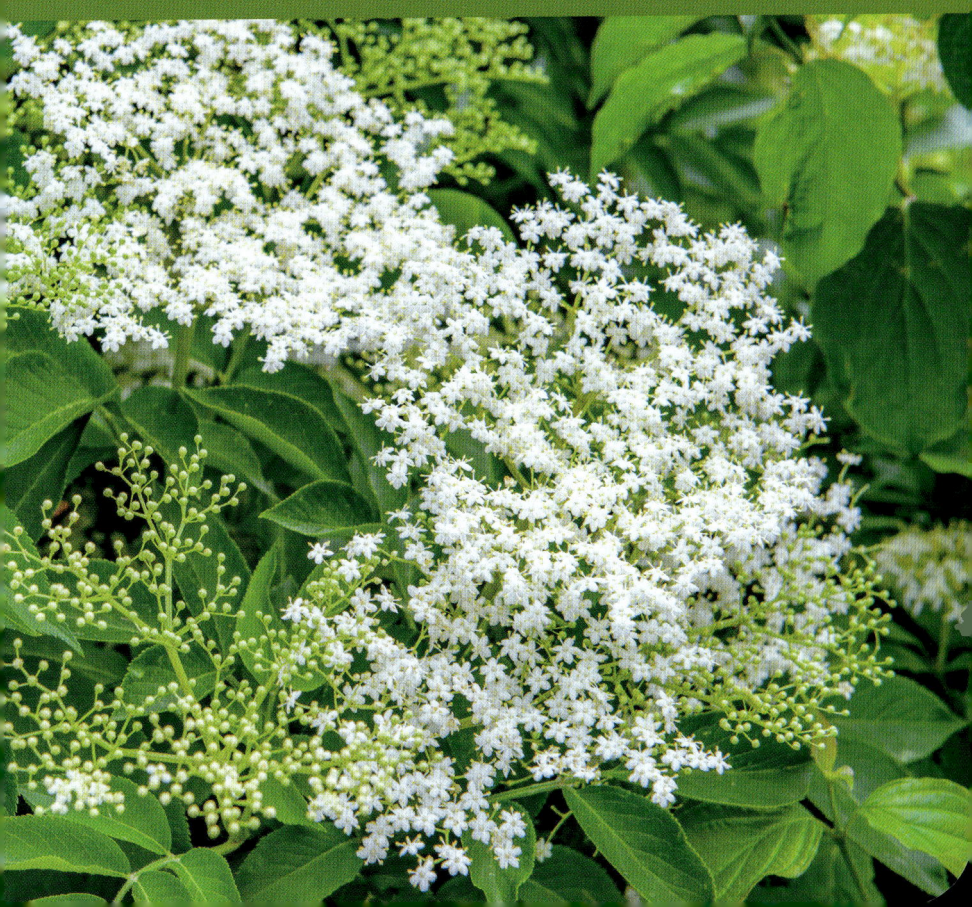

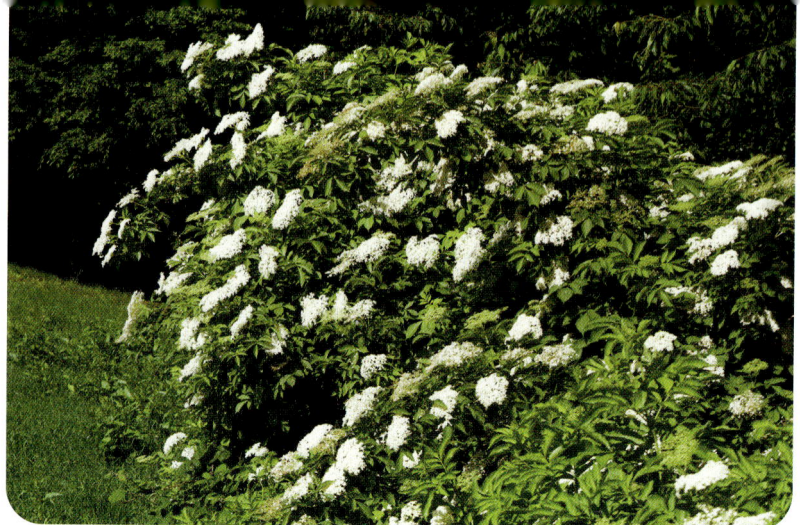

Elderberry is often found growing at the edges of forests and fields.

Elderberry is a beloved medicinal herb for many herbalists, and with good reason! The aromatic flowers, tart berries, and vibrant green leaves are all used medicinally, most commonly for immune support. These shrubs are often found along forest edges, waterfronts, and occasionally in open fields. They are tolerant of full to partial sun. In spring their bright white blooms are visible even from a distance. I love integrating this plant into my herbal practice because it is easy to identify in the wild, tasty, and smells lovely. I tend to work with *Sambucus nigra* and *S. canadensis,* which grow throughout eastern North America, while *S. mexicana* grows farther west and into the tropics; all three have similar medicinal properties.

BENEFITS

Immunostimulant. Stimulates immune activity

Diaphoretic. Increases sweating to break fever

Antibacterial and antimicrobial. Inhibits pathogens, bacteria, and harmful microbes

Expectorant. Aids in clearing mucus from the chest

IDENTIFICATION

Elderberry is a perennial shrub that can grow up to 10 feet tall and blooms in spring, fruiting in summer. Its compound pinnate leaves are serrated and easy to distinguish alongside the dotted bark. The dots are *lenticels*, small pores that allow gas exchange. You'll notice the dotted bark on the older stems near the ground, but the new growth will be a solid green. The white flowers grow in flat or umbrella-shaped clusters and ripen into purple berries a few months after blooming. The flower heads occur all over the plant, emerging from the new growth and tender stems.

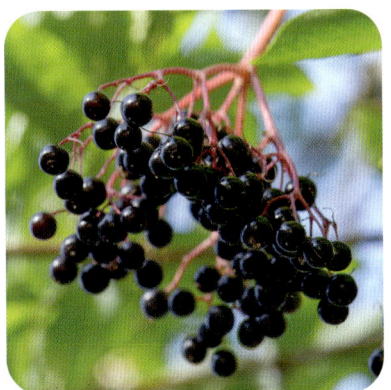

Harvest elderberries when they have darkened from red to a deep, blackish purple.

TRADITIONAL USAGE

Elderberries are used as a powerful medicine that supports the respiratory and immune systems. It's a favorite for winter herbal care and during the transition between seasons, when cold and flu symptoms abound. The flowers and berries are used most frequently for medicine.

Historically this plant has been used throughout Europe and by Indigenous peoples of the Americas. The cycles of elderberry help many tribes identify seasonal cycles in other aspects of life. For example, the northern foothill Yokut people of present-day California know that when the elderberries ripen, sugar

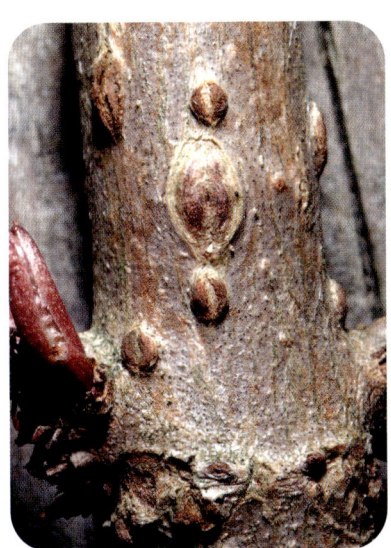

Elderberry bark is covered in small dots called lenticels.

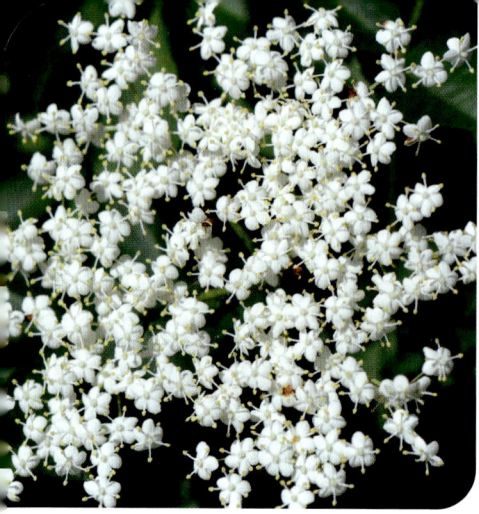

pine nuts are also ready for harvest. Similarly, coastal Pomo people on the West Coast know when to harvest shellfish based on the ripening of the rich purple elderflower berries.

Elderflowers have a unique aroma that folks either love or hate. I personally love it and opt for teas and tinctures in early summer when the blooms light up forest edges. The flowers can be used in tea to lower fevers and induce sweating. In addition to drinking the tea, Indigenous peoples of North America have also added elderflowers to baths to achieve the same purpose. Aside from lowering fever, elderflowers are used to reduce many other symptoms that accompany a cold, such as runny nose, itchy throat, and cough. Their anti-inflammatory properties make them a powerful ally for seasonal allergies, and they can help reduce swelling in the sinuses.

Elderberries arrive a few months after the first blooms. The berries provide a powerful boost to the immune system and are commonly used in tinctures, syrups, and tea blends. They are excellent for seasonal cold and flu symptoms and for respiratory conditions. I always keep some dried and ready during winter. They're best taken as soon as you feel symptoms begin. Overall, elderberries are a powerful ally for any illness, a great immune boost, and an ideal tonic for winter wellness.

HARVESTING

Elderberries typically bloom in late spring or early summer. They will develop fruit by midsummer into early fall. When harvesting elderflowers or berries, cut at the base of the cluster, right before the leaves begin. This plant loves to grow in transitional spaces, especially in disturbed areas, so be mindful of any kind of soil pollution, industrial sites, or polluted waterways nearby. To prevent the fragile flowers or berries from being crushed, use a collection container, such as a bucket or even a paper shopping bag to provide some structure and protection. Elderberries are ripe when they are a dark blackish purple, with no trace of red on the berry, and can be easily crushed. You may even see birds fly away as you approach, signifying they've begun their harvest as well.

PREPARATION

Elderberries can be dried or frozen for use during the winter season. To make a healing decoction, you can boil the fresh berries for 5 to 10 minutes, until the water turns a rich color. Try adding aromatic spices, such as cinnamon and ginger, which can help with cold and flu symptoms. Dried berries make an excellent infusion.

Elderflowers are fragile and aromatic and work well in infusions. They're excellent infused into honey to make a medicinal sweetener. My favorite ways to prepare elderflowers are to harvest them fresh and use them for tea, make a sweet vegetable glycerin tincture, or make a simple syrup. Elderflower syrups are often commercially available, but you can make your own by simmering the flowers in water and sugar (see page 244). The flowers can also be dried and preserved for later use. But keep in mind that if you harvest the flowers, you won't get any berries.

Elderberry leaves can be made into a decoction by boiling for 5 to 10 minutes; try adding some honey since the bitter green flavor can be strong.

Process Before Snacking

Elderberries can be eaten raw in small amounts, but excessive snacking can cause stomach upset. Err on the side of caution and boil berries before use.

ELDERBERRY FAST FACTS

- Leaves are compound pinnate and serrated
- Commonly found on forest edges and alongside water
- Woody stem covered in lenticels, small brown dots
- Flowers and berries grow in a cluster (flat or rounded), sometimes drooping downward
- One main stem or multiple shoots emerging from soil; newest growth is light green in color
- White flowers, leaves, and ripe berries used medicinally; always cook berries before consuming

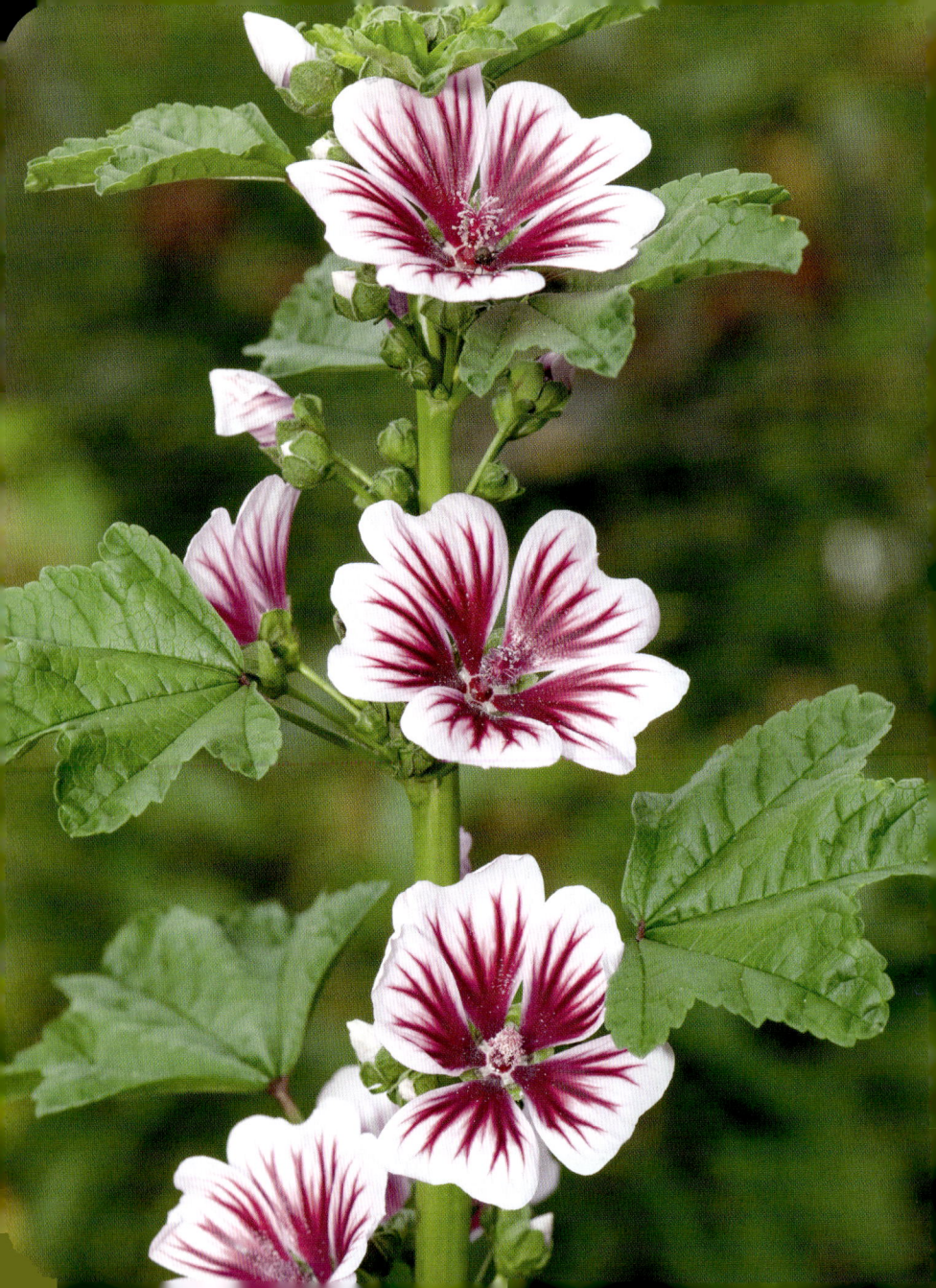

MALLOW

Malva sylvestris
Family: Malvaceae

Other Names: cheeses, high mallow

Parts Used: leaves and fruits

When to Harvest: spring and summer

Wild mallows are a group of plants in the mallow family (crazy, right?), also called Malvaceae. Other plants in this family include okra (*Abelmoschus esculentus*), hibiscus (*Hibiscus sabdariffa*), cotton (*Gossypium* spp.), and jute (*Corchorus olitorius*). If you've ever eaten raw okra, you know it's uniquely slimy. The slime is due to mucilage, a polysaccharide-rich substance found in plants that often have a cooling and moistening effect on the body. Mallow is rich in mucilage, making its leaves and seeds beautifully slimy. Sometimes called *cheeses* because their seeds resemble wheels of cheese, many species of mallow have naturalized in the Americas, and they often grow in yards and disturbed areas.

BENEFITS

Demulcent. Cooling and soothing

Diuretic. Helps the body eliminate excess water through increased urination

Expectorant. Aids in clearing mucus from the chest

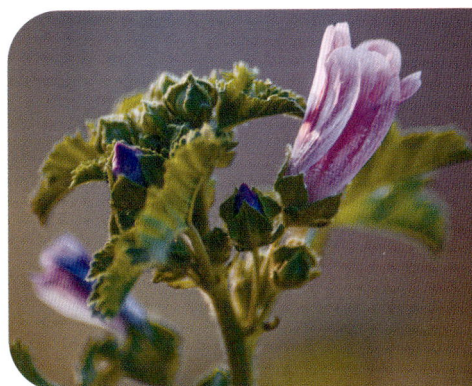

The best time to harvest mallow is when it has begun to develop flower buds but before they open.

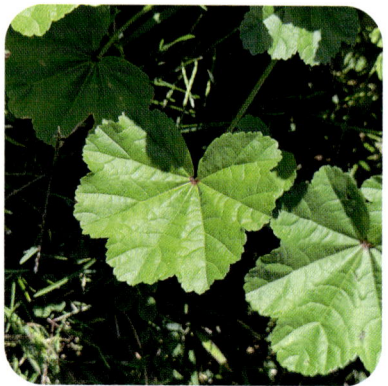
Harvest mallow leaves when they're fully developed but not overly fibrous.

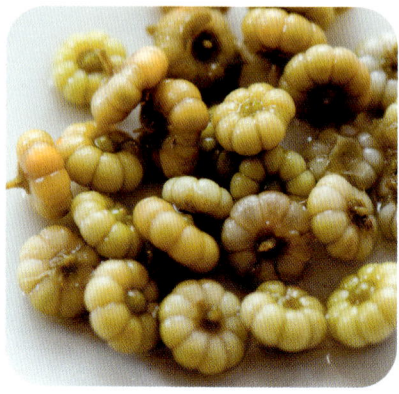
Mallow fruits look like tiny wheels of cheese, earning these plants the nickname "cheeses."

IDENTIFICATION

Mallow is a common plant, often popping up in garden beds and yards. If you ever pull one up, you'll notice a very long taproot, which makes them notoriously hard to eliminate. The leaves, basal with five to seven distinct, shallow lobes, can be kidney-shaped or rounded and are fuzzy. The leaves grow erect later in the season before flowering. The single-stemmed flowers bloom white to purple, depending on the variety. The fruits, which emerge after the flowers are pollinated, look like cheese wheels with little concentric circles at their centers, and can be up to an inch in size. This plant is a perennial and can grow up to a foot tall at its peak height.

TRADITIONAL USAGE

Used throughout Asia, Europe, and Africa, mallow has long been prized for its mucilage. The mucilage is cooling and soothing for digestive system irritation, easing ulcer pain, cooling down the heat resulting from eating too much spicy food, and addressing other gut issues. The leaves can be eaten or made into tea for this purpose.

Mallow is a mild diuretic, helping move water within the body, and has been used for ailments such as edema and other forms of excessive water retention. As an expectorant, the mucilage in mallow helps loosen phlegm and congestion and accelerates the healing process.

HARVESTING

When harvesting the leaves, aim for the sweet spot between a small, newly unfurled leaf and an older, overly fibrous leaf. The ideal time to harvest is when the plant is growing erect and will soon be sending out flower buds. Harvest plants that are growing upright and not on the ground, as those can sometimes be covered in various types of fungus. Harvest the entire leaf, petiole and all. If harvesting fruits, pick when they are green and fresh, rubbing them between your hands to separate the fruit from the calyx and cluster.

PROCESSING

Have you ever cooked okra and noticed that after enough boiling or sautéing, the slime is gone? That's because mucilage is sensitive to heat and too much will destroy it. Mallow works best in water-based preparations, and since mallow mucilage is our friend, it's best extracted using what's called a *cold infusion*. See page 211 for details on how to make one. Mallow makes a refreshing and nourishing preparation, especially in summertime. Preparations like this are usually drunk the same day, as they are prone to molding, particularly if the plant material is fresh.

Mallow leaves tend to dry very easily. If you have fruits you'd like to dry, it's best to use a dehydrator, as they are slimy and dense. Consider slicing them in half to speed the drying process. The fresh fruits can also be used or eaten raw; they are rich in the same mucilage that makes the leaves demulcent and medicinal.

MALLOW FAST FACTS

- Leaves are basal, growing erect later in season before blooming
- Kidney-shaped or round leaves are fuzzy with five to seven distinct and shallow lobes
- When fruiting, fruit resembles cheese wheel (circular with a smaller concentric circle within)
- If uprooted, you'll notice a long taproot
- White to purple flowers
- Commonly growing in grass and on walkways, but can grow along forest edges

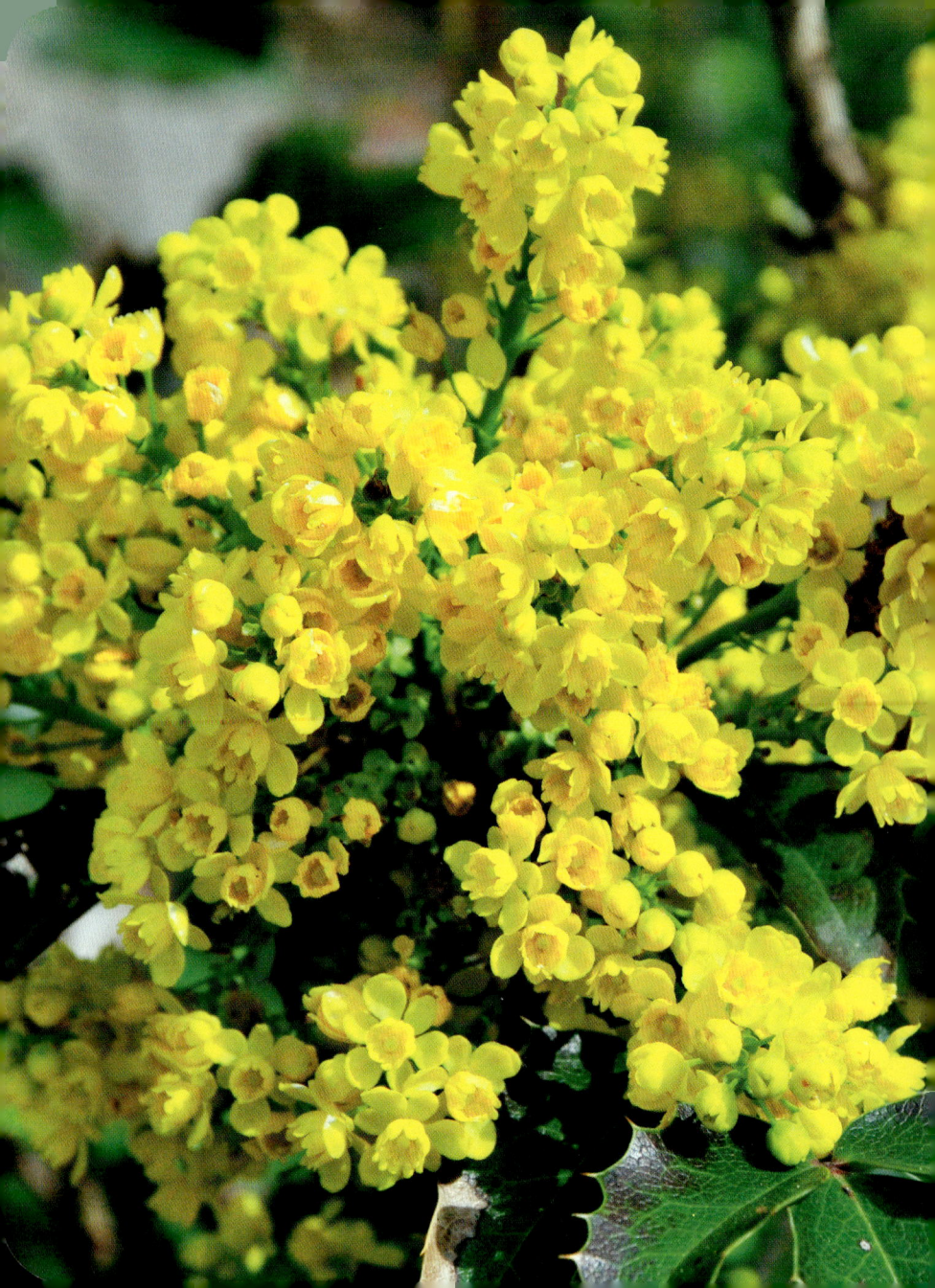

CHAPTER 6

Forest MEDICINE

The plants discussed in this chapter are all forest dwellers. Venturing into the peace of the woods is a restorative experience in and of itself, but encountering these healing plants makes it even better.

BLACK WALNUT

Juglans nigra
Family: Juglandaceae

Other Names: American black walnut

Parts Used: leaves, unripe and ripe hull of fruits, and nuts

When to Harvest: fall

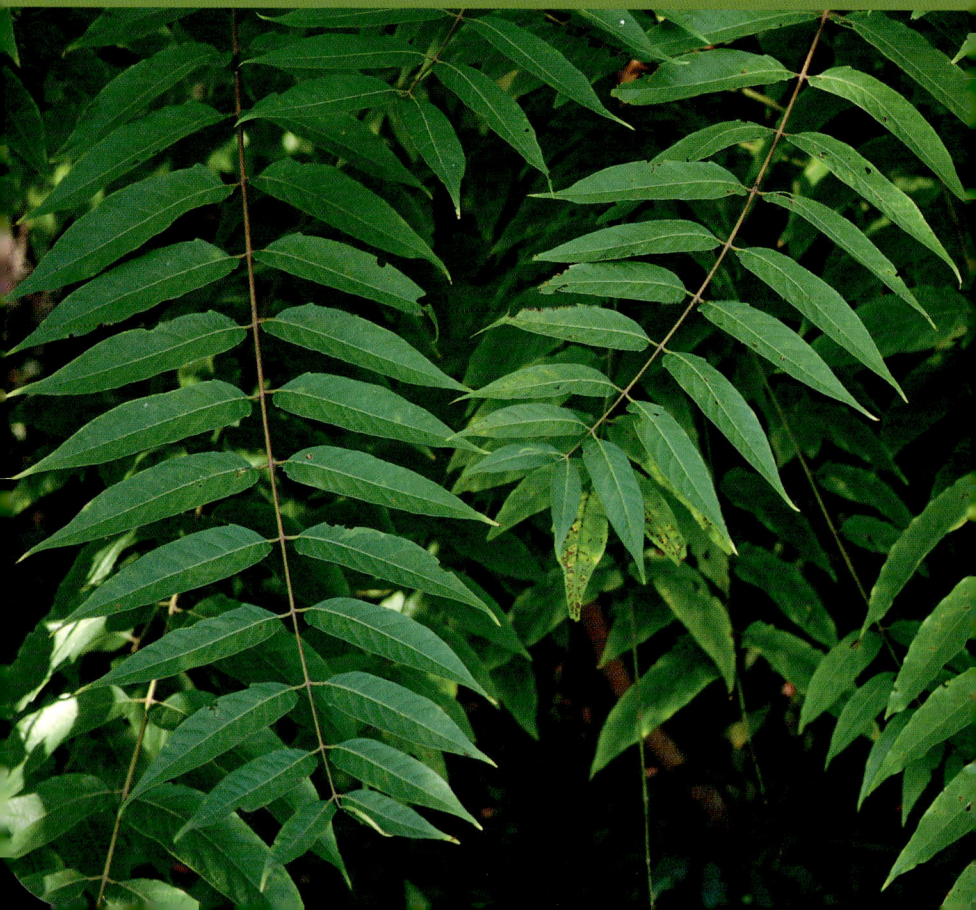

Black walnuts covered the roadsides and riverbeds around the Carolinas where I grew up, and staining my hands collecting these nuts was one of my favorite pastimes as a very young herbalist. The delicious walnuts inside made the hours of smashing and cracking shells worth it. A native tree common throughout the East to the Midwest, black walnut has been a staple of Indigenous foods, medicines, and textiles for thousands of years. It remains a prominent plant in many herbalists' medicine cabinets.

BENEFITS

Antiparasitic. Inhibits parasitic organisms

Antifungal. Inhibits fungal growth

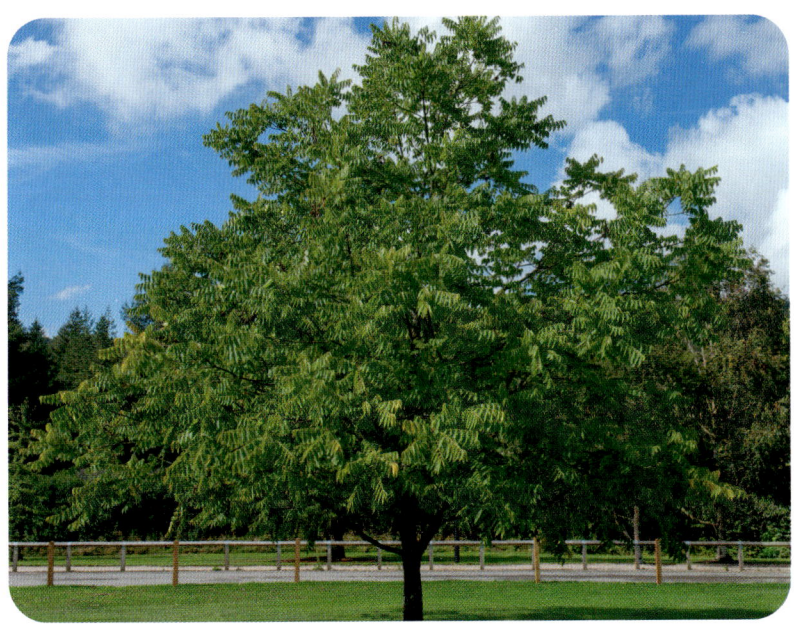

Indigenous people have long used black walnut as a food staple and powerful medicine.

IDENTIFICATION

Black walnut is a large tree with distinct ridges in its bark. The leaves are large and compound and have up to 23 leaflets arranged in opposite pairs. The fuzzy new growth is a vibrant green color that turns to yellow in fall. Green fruits develop through summer into fall, growing in clusters and eventually falling to the ground when ripe. The fruits are composed of a firm hull wrapped around the hard nut, with the edible nutmeat inside. When unripe, the fruit is whitish yellow inside, but as it ripens it turns a dark brown that stains the skin. The fruit has a distinctly spicy citrus aroma when scratched, as do the leaves when crushed.

TRADITIONAL USAGE

Unripe and ripe black walnut hulls (the outer layer surrounding the shell of the nut) can be boiled and drunk as a remedy to intestinal parasites and worms. In my experience, parasite cleanses can be overemphasized, so it's best to be sure of what is happening in your body before taking this plant in high doses. It can be irritating and even damaging to the system to take large or consistent doses of plants that are antifungal or antiparasitic. Always seek expert advice.

As an antifungal, the hulls are boiled and the liquid is used to wash skin affected by ailments such as ringworm and athlete's foot. The leaves are occasionally used as well but are considered less potent than the hull. The bark has historically been employed medicinally, but it contains some toxic compounds that can irritate the digestive system with long-term use, so it's best to use the hulls instead.

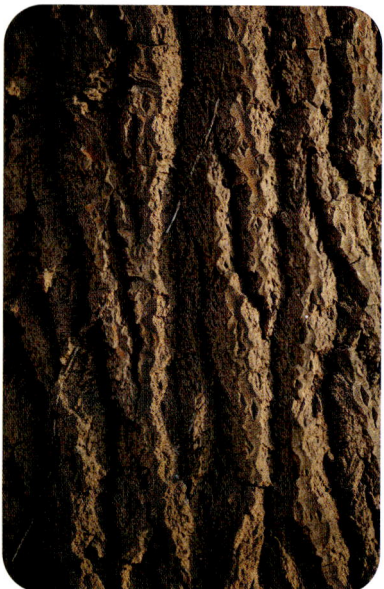

The bark of the black walnut is distinctively ridged.

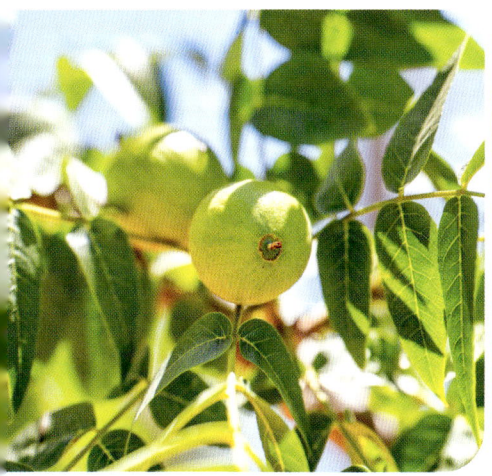 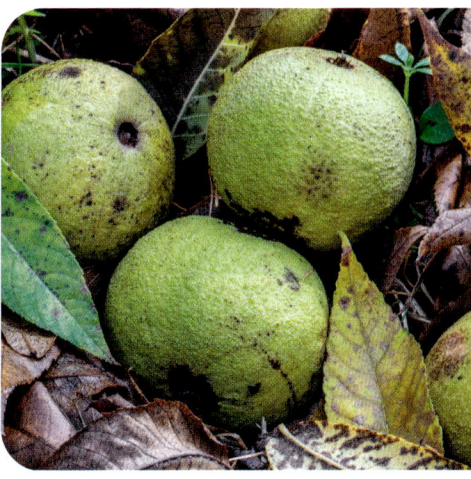

Black walnut is ideally harvested directly from the tree when it's slightly underripe, but that can be difficult depending on the size of the tree. When gathering windfall fruit, look for fruit with a green exterior that is still firm.

HARVESTING

Black walnut is medicinal when ripe but is considered more potent when unripe. Harvest in early to mid-fall when the fruits are two to three inches in diameter. Black walnuts are large trees, which can make reaching the unripe fruit a little bit tricky. A tree with low branches is ideal if you can find one. If the fruit is inaccessible you can wait until it has ripened and fallen to the ground. It will sometimes fall off the tree before maturing, so check often. If you're gathering windfall fruit, collect it soon after it falls, as you'll see worms starting to eat the inner hull on older fruit. Look for fruit that is green, aromatic, and semifirm, instead of completely browned or mushy.

The hull is very easy to separate from the nut with a hammer. To use the nuts, simply separate them from the hulls, clean off any residue, and leave them in a well-ventilated space for a few weeks before opening the shells with a hammer or nutcracker to access the edible center.

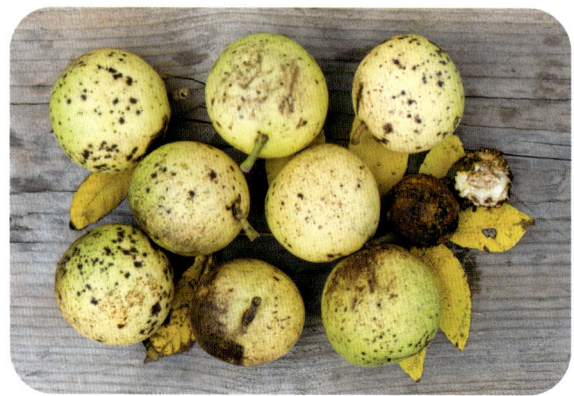

The hull of the fruit, which surrounds the nut in the center, has the most medicinal qualities.

BLACK WALNUT FAST FACTS

- In fall, check concrete or ground below the tree for fallen fruit or brown-stained sidewalks
- Large, compound leaves with up to 23 leaflets
- Newest stem growth is fuzzy in contrast to woody branches and bark
- Clusters of green fruit growing to the size of a baseball
- When scraped, fruits emit strong, spicy citrus aroma
- Fruit is best harvested unripe or when ripe but still firm

PREPARATION

Black walnut can be made into tea, but I've found the flavor is unappealing and it will stain if it spills. Instead, try tincturing black walnut hull for acute usage. This can be done with the fresh or dried hulls. A few hits from a hammer will separate the hull from the nut inside. Softer, slightly mushy (but still green fruit) can even be separated with your hands. If you want to dry the hulls, crush them well and leave them in the sun, put them in a dehydrator, or even dry them on a very low setting (see page 50) in the oven. Once they're dry, they can be easily ground into powder and stored for later use.

STINGING NETTLE

Urtica dioica
Family: Urticaceae

Other Names: common nettle, burn nettle

Parts Used: leaves, shoots, seeds, and roots

When to Harvest: spring and fall

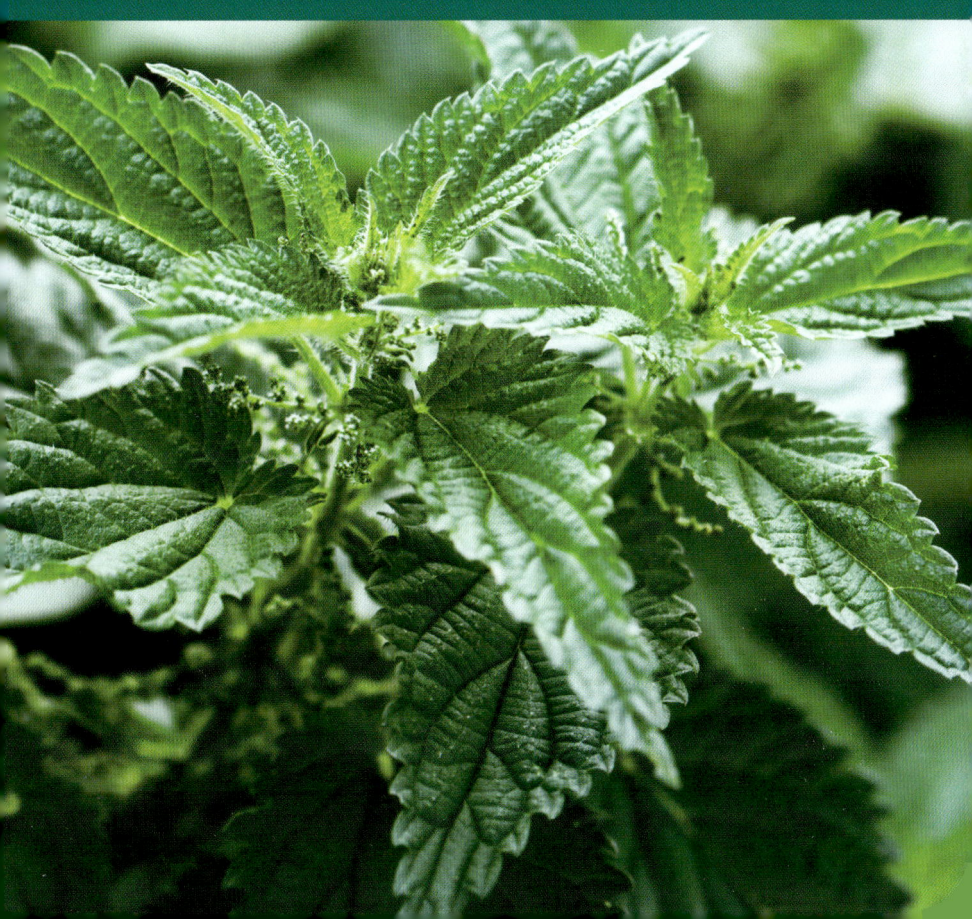

A friend to herbalists and a foe to others, stinging nettle is one of our greatest plant allies. A nutritive and stinging wonder, it is originally native to Europe and has naturalized in temperate climates around the world. Many places have a local version of nettle, such as *Urera baccifera,* native to tropical regions, or *Laportea canadensis* in North America; they tend to be used very similarly to the stinging nettle (*Urtica dioica*) described here. Whether boiled in tea, cooked as a green, or accidentally brushed against in the forest, nettle is unforgettable!

BENEFITS

Nutritive. Rich in vitamins and minerals

Diuretic. Helps the body eliminate excess water through increased urination

Anti-inflammatory. Eases inflammation

General wellness tonic.

IDENTIFICATION

Nettle plants can grow between one and four feet tall and are well adapted to various types of soil. Nettle's leaves are opposite and run up the stem, with the newest growth at the top. Its leaves tend to be dark green, with a rough, hairy texture, and are serrated with a

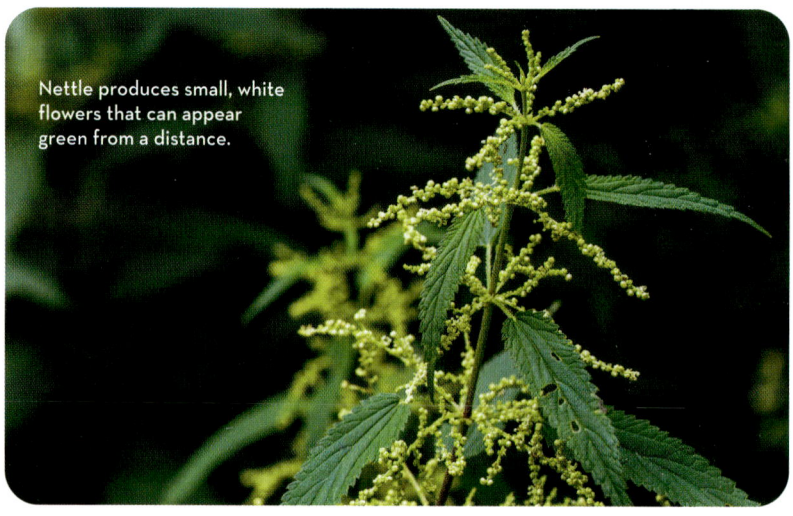

Nettle produces small, white flowers that can appear green from a distance.

rounded base and pointed end. Most of the stinging hairs are located on the square, fibrous stem. The seeds and flowers are long and hairy, emerging from the top 12 inches of the stem at the leaf nodes. The flowers look green from afar, but upon close examination you can see the tiny white blooms. Not sure if it's nettle? You can always touch it and find out!

TRADITIONAL USAGE

Stinging nettle is a powerful nutritive medicine. Rich in protein, calcium, trace minerals, iron, and various vitamins, nettle's nourishing properties are best absorbed in an overnight infusion or by cooking and eating the new shoots. The leaves can also be made into a tea to ease the inflammation associated with allergic rhinitis, stuffy nose, and seasonal allergies. It's a common medicine to take in early spring when the plant's fresh shoots first emerge. For urinary tract irritation and excess retention of water in the body, nettle can be taken as a powerful diuretic.

Fresh stinging nettle is sometimes cut and intentionally applied to the body in areas with poor circulation, arthritis, or pain; this process is called *urtication*. The stinging sensation brings blood to the surface, resulting in itchy, red spots that ease after 20

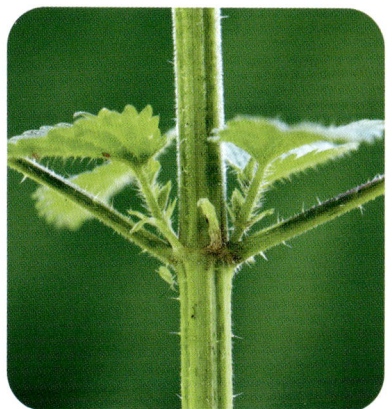

Small stinging hairs grow along nettle's square stem.

to 30 minutes for most individuals. This helps improve blood flow to areas suffering from pain and arthritis, such as the knees, hands, and joints. Nettle leaf is also used topically as a salve or wash for the hair and scalp, promoting hair growth and helping relieve ailments such as eczema and psoriasis.

Nettle roots are commonly chopped and boiled, and the decoction is taken internally to ease symptoms of benign prostatic hyperplasia, such as painful urination and inability to urinate. Nettle seeds are powerfully nourishing to the kidneys and body overall; they can be eaten, or they can be drunk by grinding them into powder and mixing it directly in water.

When Nettle Bites Back

If you happen to get stung by nettle while harvesting or processing, the pain and itching will generally subside within 30 minutes, but small welts may remain on your skin. If it continues to bother you, an application of calamine lotion, soothing salve, or plantain poultice (see page 230) can help ease the irritation.

HARVESTING

When harvesting nettle, it's best to wear thick gloves. Clothing that protects your arms and legs might also be helpful if you're very sensitive. To harvest the leaves, cut halfway down the stem at a leaf node and strip the leaves off the stem (which is rich in fiber, but not as useful for medicine). Nettle leaf is best harvested when the plant isn't flowering or giving seed. Nettle leaves develop higher amounts of calcium oxalates when flowering, which can be irritating to the kidneys and bladder over long periods of time. Be sure to harvest your nettle in a clean area, as it's capable of pulling up compounds such as lead from polluted soils.

The seeds can be harvested when green and dried before using. The roots can be cut into small pieces and dried for future use. Fresh shoots for cooking tend to be the best and most tender in early spring or fall.

PREPARATION

Making an overnight infusion of stinging nettle is one of my favorite ways to work with this plant (see page 210). The result is a dark green, almost black infusion, rich in vitamins and minerals, that will support you throughout the day. Fresh nettle shoots are also an excellent way to consume this plant; simply steam your newly harvested, tender shoots before eating. After being lightly cooked, the shoots are great anywhere you would add other types of greens—in pesto or soup or simply alone with onions and garlic. Nettle seeds can be eaten raw or added to any recipe for baking. Many people like to dry the seeds before using them in this way, as it results in a flourlike consistency; however, the fresh seeds can also be added. The fresh or dried roots can be boiled and drunk as tea or made into a tincture.

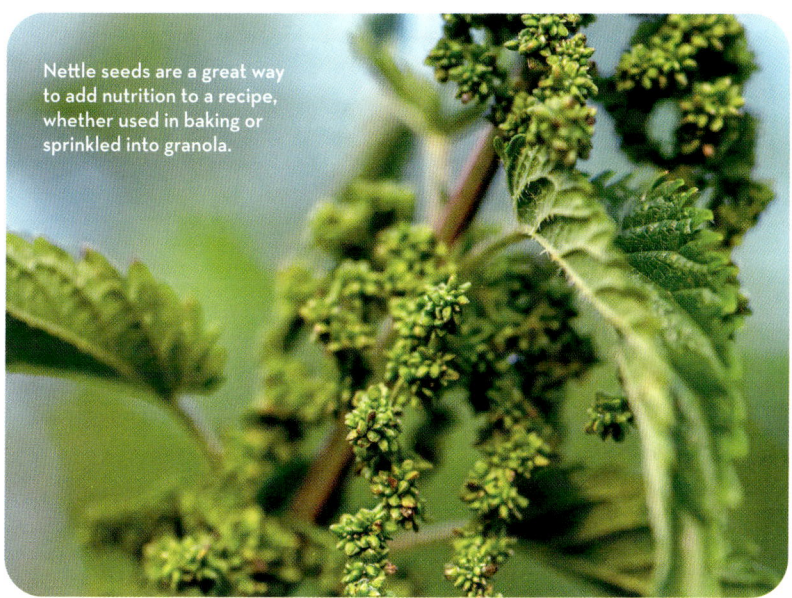

Nettle seeds are a great way to add nutrition to a recipe, whether used in baking or sprinkled into granola.

STINGING NETTLE FAST FACTS

- Opposite leaves with a rough, hairy texture
- Fine, stinging hairs along entire plant
- Leaves have a rounded base with serrated edges, dark green color
- Seed clusters develop near new growth, will drop off plant later in the season
- Best to harvest leaves before the plant goes to seed in spring or early fall
- Leaves, seeds, shoots, and roots are all used

OREGON GRAPE

Mahonia aquifolium
Family: Berberidaceae

Other Names: Oregon grape holly

Parts Used: roots, stem, and bark

When to Harvest: spring and fall

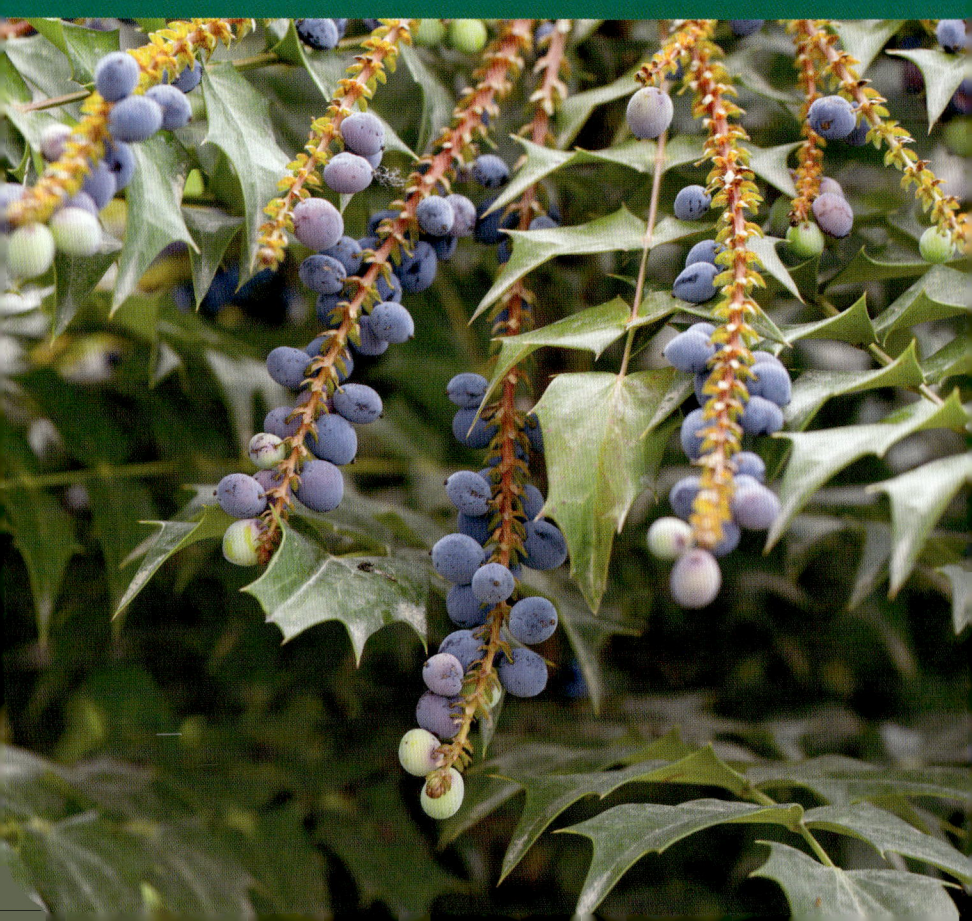

Despite its name, Oregon grape doesn't only grow in Oregon. A commonly landscaped plant, Oregon grape is native to western North America but is considered invasive even in parts of the Southeast. This plant is a small shrub, growing five to six feet at most, with showy blue berries during its fruiting cycle. The spiky leaves, reminiscent of holly, stand out in the forest. While the fruits are occasionally used for food, it's the roots that are primarily used as a powerful medicine. Rich in an alkaloid called *berberine*, this plant is an amazing ally that can stand in for goldenseal (*Hydrastis canadensis*), which has similar compounds but is endangered in eastern North America.

BENEFITS

Antimicrobial. Inhibits microbial growth

Antibacterial. Inhibits bacterial growth

Astringent. Tonifies skin and smooth muscle tissue

IDENTIFICATION

Oregon grape is a small shrub growing three to six feet tall with green, glossy leaves. The leaves are compound pinnate with 7 to 10 leaflets. They are very firm and have spikes along the wavy edges. The thick stems are woody and tend to grow in clusters from the roots. When blooming, large bunches of bright yellow flowers emerge at the top of

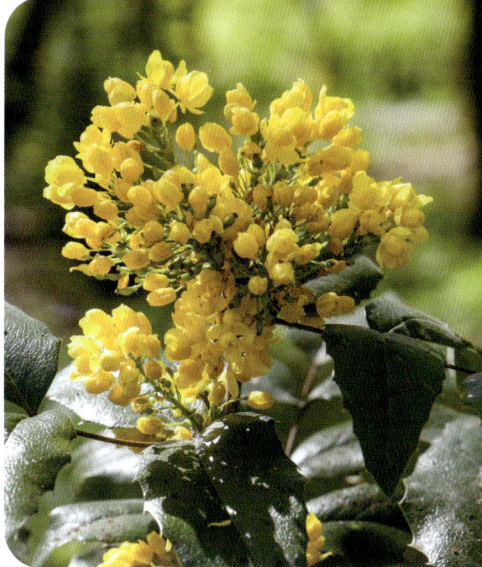

The yellow flowers of Oregon grape will develop into bright blue fruit.

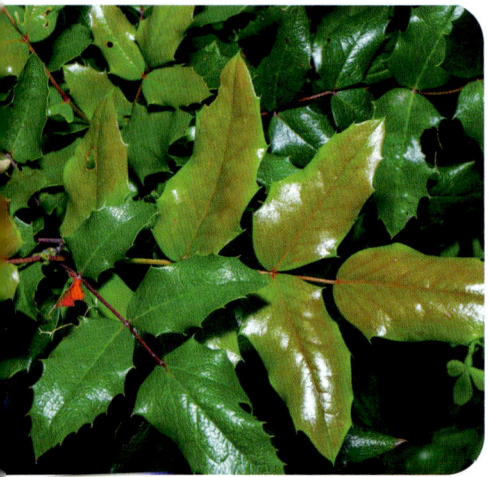

the plant, eventually turning into blue, grapelike fruits covered in powdery wild yeast. When scraped or cut, the roots and stem are a vibrant yellow inside, characteristic of many plants containing berberine.

TRADITIONAL USAGE

Oregon grape can be used as a powerful antibiotic, antimicrobial, and astringent thanks to berberine, the alkaloid responsible for its bright yellow root color. The alkaloid is best extracted by making a decoction or tincture and is often used for infections in the smooth muscle tissue, such as the gums, digestive tract, and urinary tract. Various Indigenous peoples of North America also use this plant for lowering fevers and as a dye for textiles. The bitter flavor of berberine helps the digestive system, stimulating digestion and helping relieve constipation.

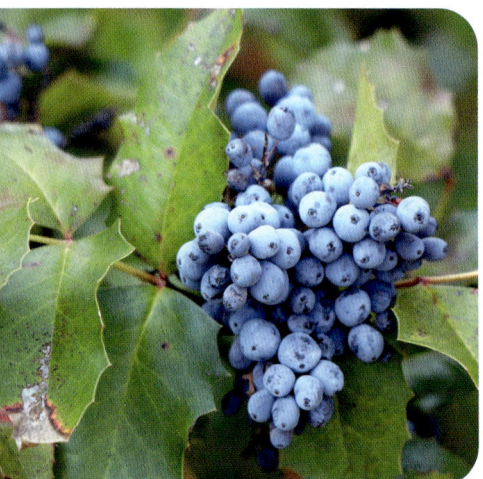

The leaves of Oregon grape can look glossy on the top, a helpful identifying feature.

Avoid If Pregnant

Due to the berberine content in this plant, Oregon grape should not be taken during pregnancy.

HARVESTING

Before you harvest, it's important to consider the status of the plant wherever you are located. As always, avoid harvesting this plant in places where it is at risk. On the West Coast of North America, this plant is considered at risk in the wild. On the East Coast, however, it is considered invasive and spreads quickly, shading out native plants in the forest.

The roots, bark, and stem are best gathered after the fruit drops. Avoid harvesting the plant when it's blooming or fruiting, as the plant's energy will be focused on the flowers and fruit at that time. You'll need a shovel and sharp knife to harvest this plant, especially if digging up the roots that sprawl out under the soil.

PROCESSING

Since the roots and stem are often quite thick, it's best to chop this plant well to allow it to dry evenly. Try to do this within a day of harvesting, as it will become more difficult to cut as it dries. Fresh roots and bark can be made into a tincture. That is one of my favorite ways to use this medicine, as it minimizes the bitter taste and works more acutely when administered.

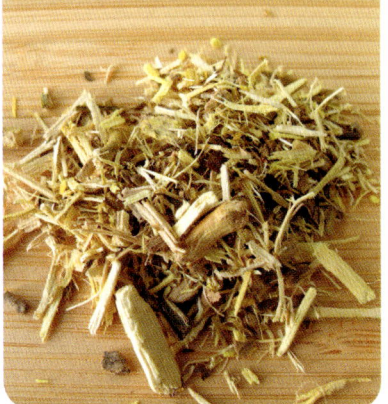

The roots of Oregon grape are full of berberine, which gives them a bright yellow color.

OREGON GRAPE FAST FACTS

- Glossy compound pinnate leaves with sharp, spiky edges
- Three- to six-foot-tall plant
- Roots or stem can be cut to reveal bright yellow color inside, caused by berberine
- Bright yellow flower clusters turn into blue, grapelike fruits covered in powdery wild yeast
- In western North America, be cautious when harvesting, as plant is considered at risk; in eastern North America it's considered invasive
- Roots and stem best harvested after fruits drop; fruits are edible but not medicinal

BEE BALM

Monarda spp. (*M. didyma*, *M. punctata*)
Family: Lamiaceae

Other Names: Oswego tea, bergamot

Parts Used: leaves and flower heads

When to Harvest: summer

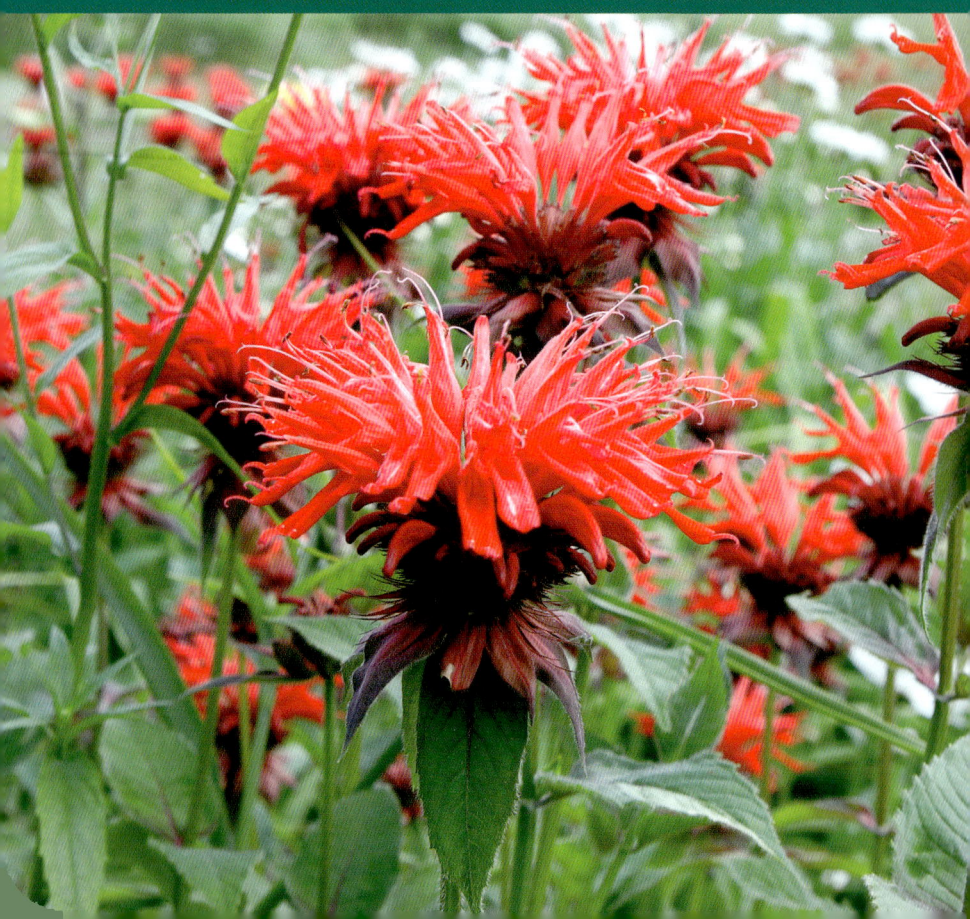

Blooming in fields, along roadsides, and in many gardens, bee balm is a colorful addition to the landscape. Rich in aromatic oils, this warming medicine has long been used throughout North America by Indigenous peoples. Commonly called *wild oregano* by the Gullah Geechee people of Lowcountry South Carolina and beyond, the thymol-rich leaves give off a spicy aroma reminiscent of thyme or oregano.

BENEFITS

Carminative. Enhances digestion

Antibacterial. Inhibits bacterial growth

Febrifuge. Lowers fevers

Decongestant. Reduces nasal congestion

IDENTIFICATION

There are a few colors of bee balm; typically, they are red, purple, pink, or one of the shades in between. They range in height from one to five feet tall, depending on the variety and species. *Monarda didyma*, commonly called scarlet bee balm, is a native perennial that grows up to five feet tall, whereas *M. punctata* (possibly my favorite

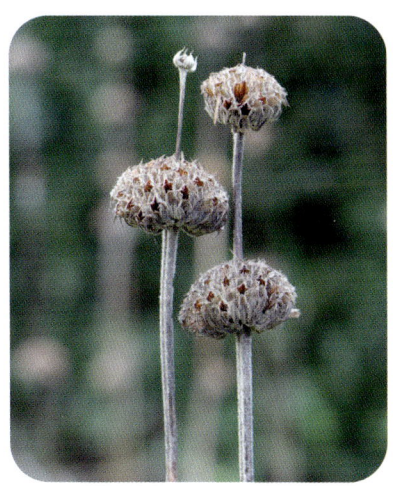

Bee balm seedpods often linger on the plant into winter.

species; don't tell the other ones) grows just one foot and is decorated with spots and pink hues. Regardless of the species, they can all be used medicinally, and their colorful blooms appear in summer. The long, tubular petals are whorled around the flower head, which appears at the top of the plant. The square stem has opposite leaves that are lanceolate and serrated, typical for a plant in the mint family. To identify bee balm when it is not in bloom, crush one of the dark green leaves and sniff for the rich, minty-oregano aroma. When the plants dry out, you'll see a large dried seed head that lingers until winter.

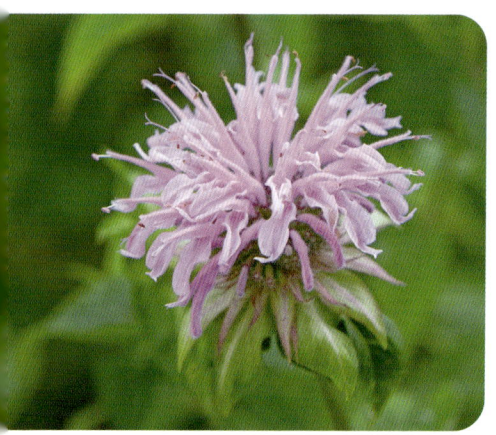

There are a variety of different species of bee balm, but they can all be used medicinally.

HARVESTING

Harvest bee balm in summer when its blooms first emerge. Cut four inches down the stem below the flowers. You can use the tender stem, leaves, and flower heads together for medicine. Harvesting early in the blooming season encourages more blooms, which means more medicine and more food for pollinators. The flowers tend to dry well if you don't want to use them immediately. I've found the flower heads are higher in aromatic and medicinal qualities than the leaves are. Be sure to harvest not only the flowers but the entire flower head, as the ball-shaped undeveloped seedpod in the center is rich in medicinal compounds when fresh.

TRADITIONAL USAGE

Bee balm has been traditionally used by Indigenous peoples of North America as both a food and a medicine. The leaves are added into various dishes to give an oregano- or thymelike flavoring; occasionally the flower heads are used for this as well. As a medicinal tea, bee balm can be used to ease sore throat, respiratory congestion, sinus infections, and digestive upset. It can also be used topically to address bacterial infections of the skin.

PREPARATION

You can prepare bee balm three primary ways: as a tea, tinctured, or in honey. Tinctures and teas extract many of the aromatic, warming qualities that make this plant valuable. When making teas, try adding a bit of honey or other warming aromatic herbs, such as sweet Annie (page 70), to complement the bee balm. As a tincture, bee balm is powerful on its own for many respiratory and cold and flu symptoms. You can even dry and powder bee balm flowers for cooking, using it as you would thyme or oregano.

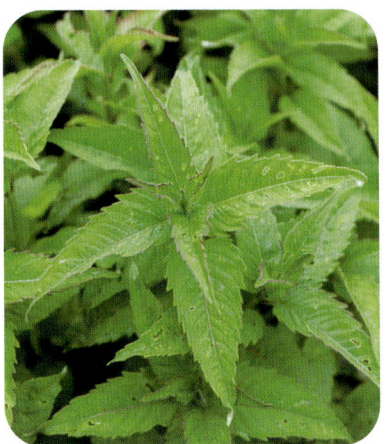

Bee balm leaves release a minty, oregano-like smell when crushed.

BEE BALM FAST FACTS

- A member of mint family; highly aromatic like oregano and thyme
- Can grow between one and five feet tall, depending on variety
- Flowers can be a wide variety of colors, including pink, purple, and red
- Purple tinge on center of leaves and on new growth
- Grows in meadows and on edges of forest
- Best harvested when in bloom, collecting whole flower heads

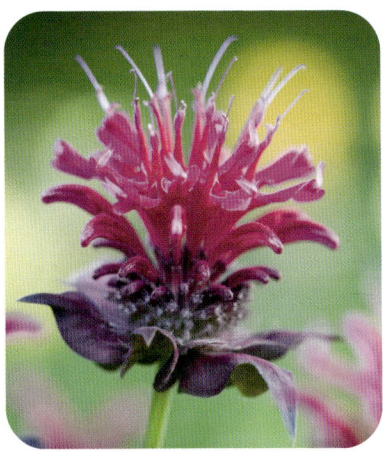

When gathering bee balm, harvest the entire flower head, as the calyx and seedpod are also medicinal.

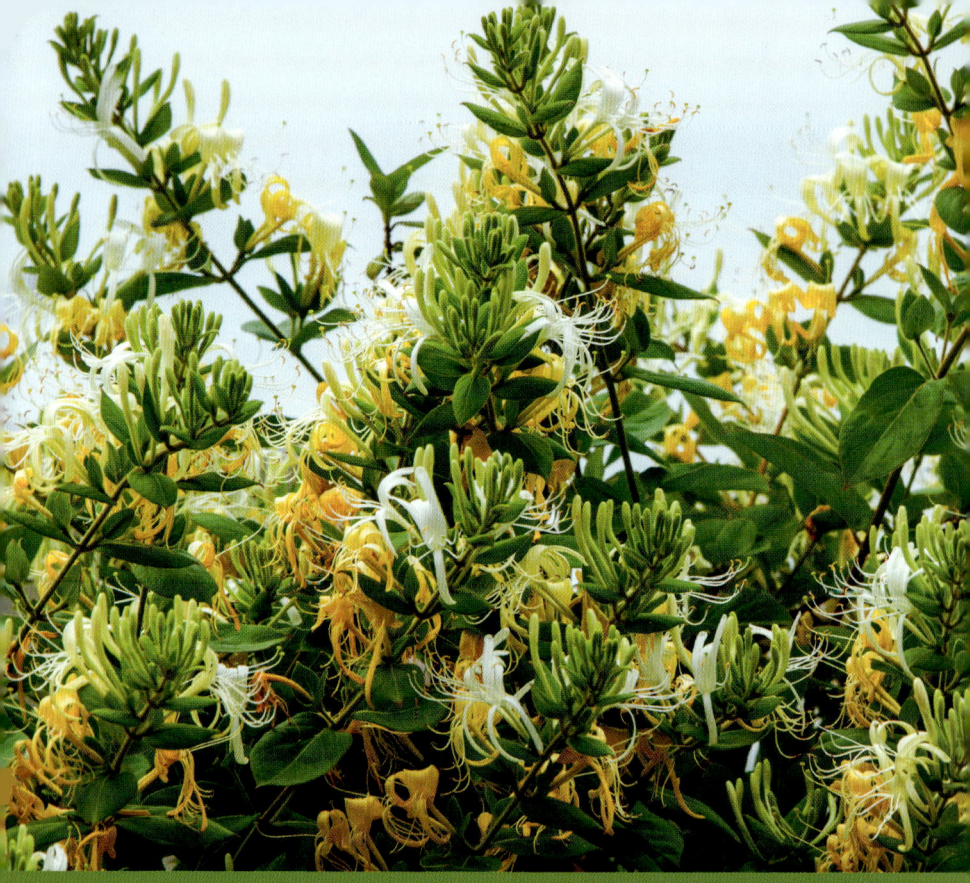

HONEYSUCKLE

Lonicera japonica
Family: Caprifoliaceae

Other Names: Japanese honeysuckle

Parts Used: flowers

When to Harvest: summer

Honeysuckle grew abundantly at the edge of the forest behind my childhood home. We would pluck the flowers as we walked, pulling them from their stems to taste the sweet drop of nectar found at the base of the flower. Though it would take hundreds of flowers to have even a mouthful of nectar, just licking a few flowers was enough to satisfy my taste buds. Take a taste the next time you see honeysuckle blooming!

Though it thrives on the forest edges in North America, honeysuckle, specifically *Lonicera japonica*, is native to Japan and is considered invasive across North America. It grows as a vine that smothers native shrubs, and it produces an abundance of white and yellow blooms.

BENEFITS

Antibacterial. Inhibits bacterial growth

Demulcent. Cooling and soothing

Antitussive. Helps stop coughing

IDENTIFICATION

Honeysuckle vine can be commonly found growing on fences, bushes, and trees in disturbed areas and gardens. The leaves are opposite and oval in shape. The top of the leaf has a slightly glossy sheen and the underside is covered with fine hairs. Newer growth has a reddish color; older growth is brown, fibrous, and woody. The white and yellow flowers grow along the vine in clusters of two to four. Blooming honeysuckle has a distinctly aromatic smell. In late summer, it will produce blackish-purple fruit that will eventually fall to the ground and germinate. The fruit is not edible.

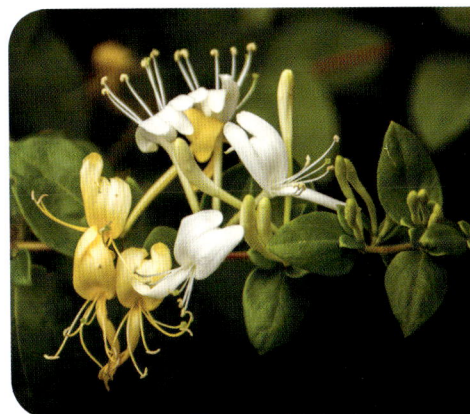

Gather honeysuckle flowers shortly after they open in order to best capture their aromatic qualities.

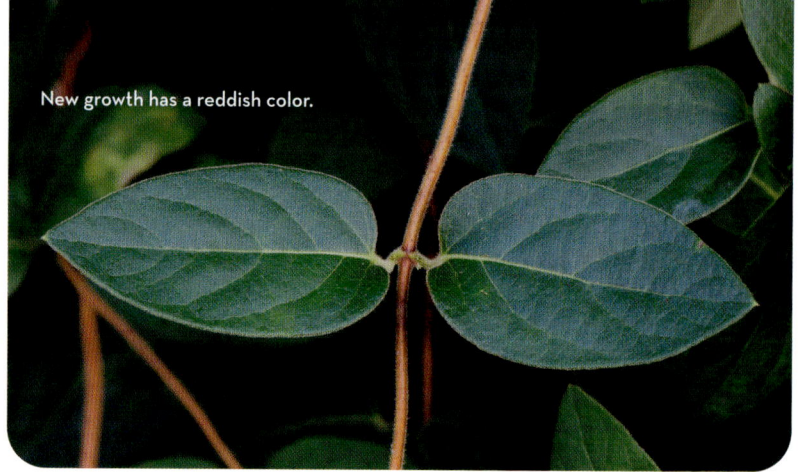

New growth has a reddish color.

TRADITIONAL USAGE

In traditional medicine throughout Asia, honeysuckle is considered a cooling, antimicrobial medicine for respiratory complaints. To use it in that way, make a strong extract either in alcohol or vegetable glycerin. You can keep the dried flowers and make infusions to ease winter colds and flu symptoms long after the blooms are gone.

The fresh flowers can be made into tea to help headaches, inflammation, and body aches. It's an excellent cooling demulcent herb, great for hot conditions such as fever, nasty coughs stemming from infection, or even excessive heat in the stomach and digestive system. It's a great way to cut the heat of summer, and in the South I've even seen it added to lemonade recipes and other refreshing drinks.

HARVESTING

Harvest blooming honeysuckle flowers throughout the year, either right as the flowers are about to open or soon after they open. To help manage this invasive plant, you can cut entire vines and bring them home to process, plucking the flowers from the vine there. Though

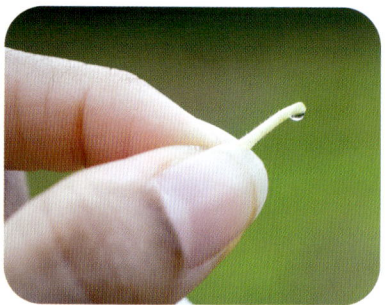

Pluck a honeysuckle flower and you'll find a single drop of sweet nectar on the end. Taste it!

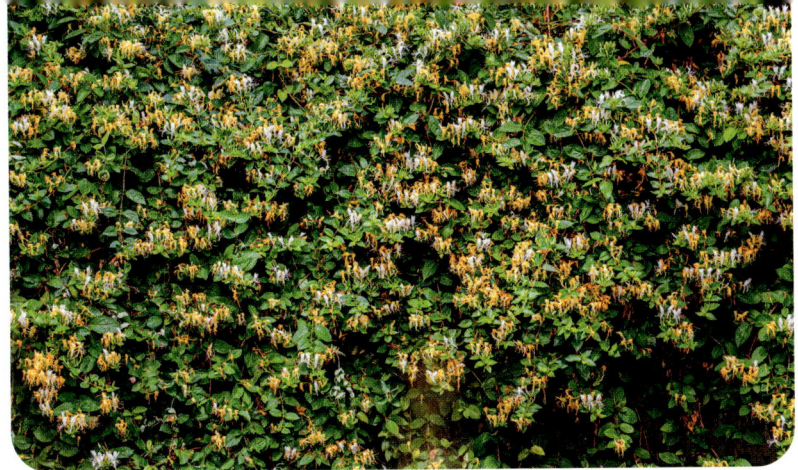

Honeysuckle can easily overwhelm native plants with its prolific growth. Cutting entire vines when you harvest it can help control its spread.

the vine's roots need to be pulled up to truly stop its growth, allowing the plants underneath it to breathe is still helpful. The flowers can be dried or used fresh. If you've harvested fresh flowers, make sure to use them within a day or two, before they wilt.

PREPARATION

Honeysuckle glycerin is an excellent way to prepare the flowers and carries the plant's aromatic qualities well. It's great for relieving issues of the respiratory system. Make a tincture, or prepare a simple tea with the crushed dried or fresh flowers; it's wonderfully aromatic and surprisingly sweet. You can also make simple syrup with the flowers, which is lovely in pastries, sodas, and more (see page 244).

HONEYSUCKLE FAST FACTS

- A vine covering shrubs, fences, and other plants; can also grow to appear like a bush
- Opposite leaves with a slightly hairy underside and a glossy top
- Stem is reddish brown at new growth, turning woody when older
- Flowers bloom in clusters of two to four and can be white or yellow
- Blackish-purple fruits at end of summer will fall off when ripe; inedible
- Flowers best harvested when in bloom in summer

RASPBERRY

Rubus idaeus, Rubus strigosus
Family: Rosaceae

Other Names: garden raspberry

Parts Used: leaves

When to Harvest: spring and late summer

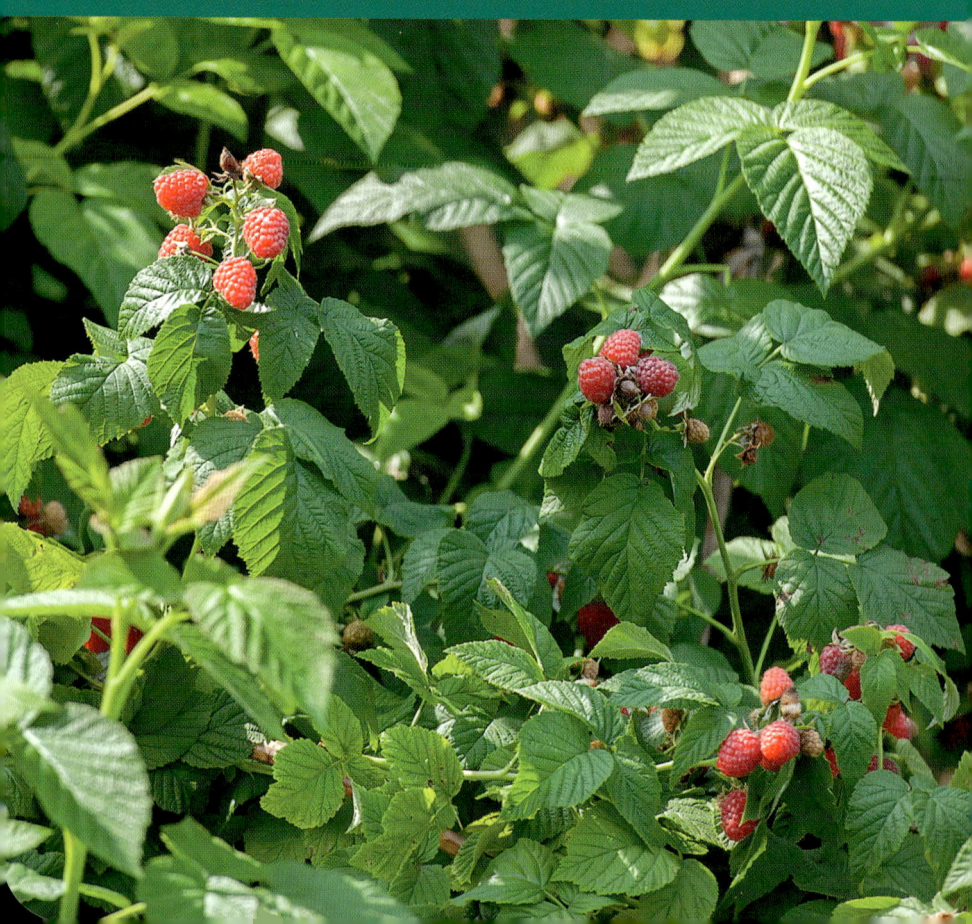

When the average person thinks of the word *raspberry*, they might imagine bright red fruit or perhaps a flavored drink. But herbalists focus on the leaves of this plant, which have a long history of medicinal usage. The fruits are easily available at any grocery store, but while they are delicious and sweet, they don't hold the same medicinal value as the leaves. Raspberry is easy to identify and is usually found at forest edges; the leaves can be harvested long after the fruit is gone. It's a medicine found in most apothecaries and is particularly helpful for menstrual health and pregnancy.

BENEFITS

Uterine tonic. Supports the uterus

Nutritive. Rich in vitamins and minerals

Astringent. Tonifies skin and smooth muscle tissue

Galactagogue. Helps increase production of breast milk

While the fruit is most familiar, raspberry leaves are actually powerfully medicinal.

IDENTIFICATION

Raspberry is a perennial bush that grows from a trailing root system; the "canes" or stems emerge from the ground anywhere along the network of roots. Other related plants, such as blackberries or dewberries, share this characteristic. The stem is covered in small spikes, with compound leaves formed from two to three leaflets. The top of the leaf is textured and green above and white or gray below.

The tell-tale sign of a red raspberry is, of course, the fruit. To avoid confusing it with an unripe blackberry, check to see if the fruit is hollow in the middle, indicating it's a raspberry, or solid, indicating

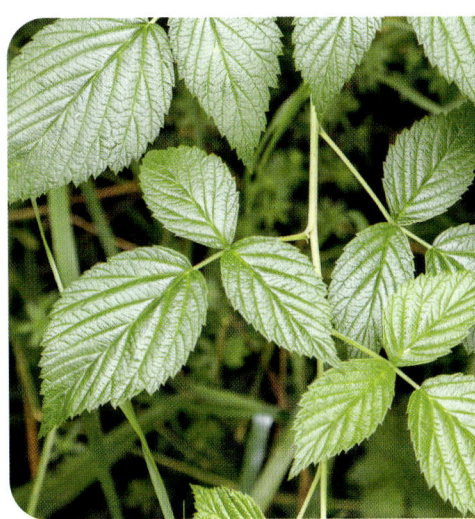

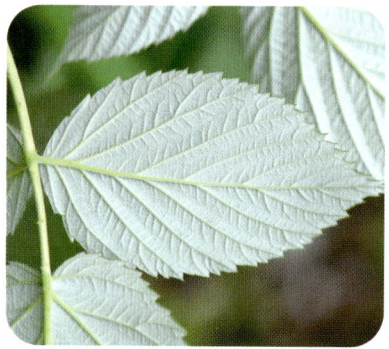

The underside of a raspberry leaf is white or gray.

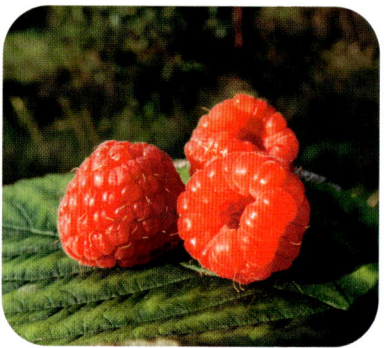

To distinguish raspberries from unripe blackberries, look for the hollow fruit.

a blackberry. *Rubus idaeus* is native to Europe and Asia and has naturalized in North America; *R. strigosus* is native to this part of the world. Both grow in similar woodside environments and can be used interchangeably.

TRADITIONAL USAGE

Raspberry's uses are numerous. It's a powerful nutritive plant, supporting the body with an abundance of vitamins and minerals, such as calcium, manganese, vitamins B and E, and even iron. It pairs well in tea with other nutritive herbs, such as stinging nettle (page 151), to fortify and invigorate the body, especially after intense events such as birth, injury, or illness.

The astringent qualities of this plant, alongside various alkaloids and phytochemicals, are beneficial to the uterus.

Raspberry leaf has traditionally been used to regulate labor contractions and ease excessive bleeding, and also to enhance the production of breast milk. Outside of pregnancy, raspberry leaf helps regulate menstrual cycles, whether bringing on menses when late, modulating irregular cycles, easing cramping, or limiting excessive bleeding. Its nourishing nutritive effect helps support the body during menstruation with iron and trace minerals. Raspberry leaf's astringency helps tonify the uterus and can ease gastrointestinal upset and irritation.

Though this plant can potentially be used at various times during pregnancy, precautions should always be taken before consuming it; consult with a healthcare provider before using.

HARVESTING

Raspberry leaves are best harvested in spring when they first emerge or in late summer, after fruiting. Gather the leaves when the plant is still putting energy into them, before they start to lose color and die off for winter. Look for leaves that are vibrant and green. You can harvest the leaves directly from the main stem, cutting close to the stem to stimulate growth.

PROCESSING

Raspberry leaves dry very easily and when crushed turn into a fluffy cluster. Simply air-dry the leaves in a well-ventilated space or put them in a dehydrator. The dried leaves can be made into a tea whenever you need a boost of nutrition or uterine support. While I typically dry raspberry leaves for future use, they can also be tinctured or made into a tea when fresh.

RASPBERRY FAST FACTS

- Leaf is textured; dark green above, grayish or white below
- Perennial emerging from canes covered in spikes
- Compound leaves with three leaflets
- If fruiting, raspberries will be hollow inside, not solid like blackberries
- Grows along forest edges in partial sun
- Leaves best harvested in early spring or after fruits have fallen off in fall

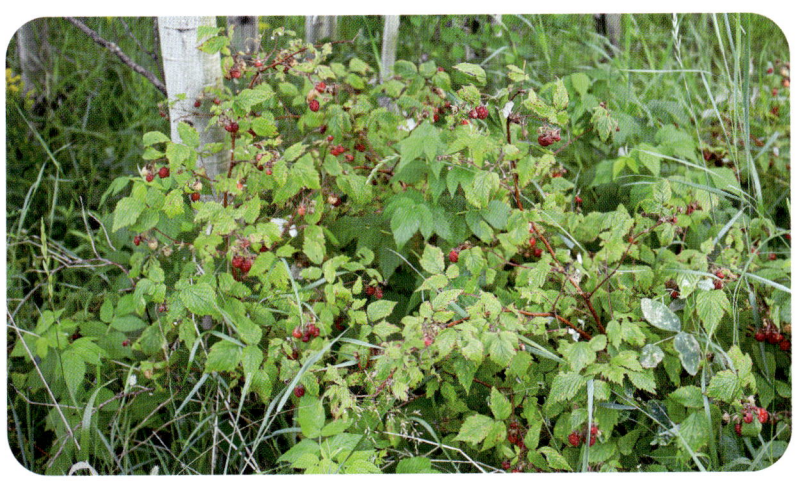

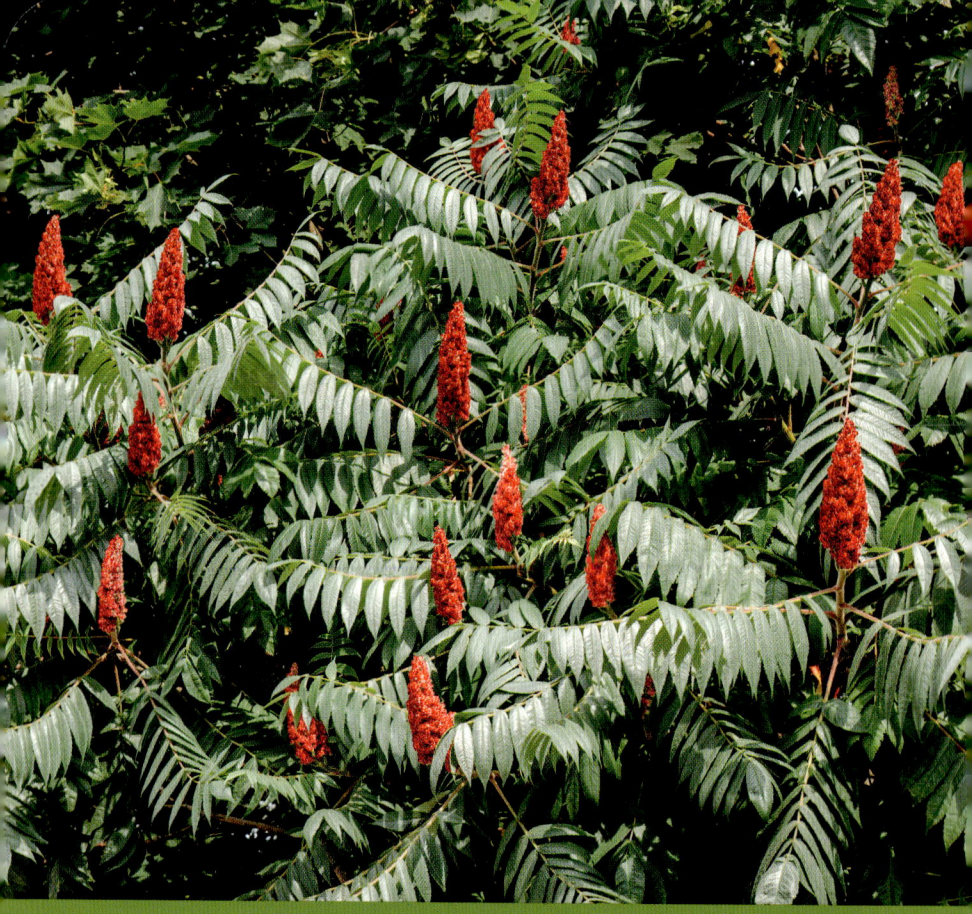

SUMAC

Rhus typhina
Family: Anacardiaceae

Other Names: staghorn sumac

Parts Used: leaves and ripe fruits

When to Harvest: summer, fall, and winter

Sumac is abundant throughout the East Coast of North America and some parts of the Midwest, with various other species growing around the world. Its fuzzy red berries turn a deep red as they mature. The berries are popularly used to make a beverage that tastes like lemonade; the high amounts of ascorbic acid make them particularly tangy and perfect for a cool drink. In addition to its culinary uses, it's a powerful medicinal plant. The plant varies in size depending on where it grows; you may see three-foot-tall plants in some areas and later drive by sumac towering over your head.

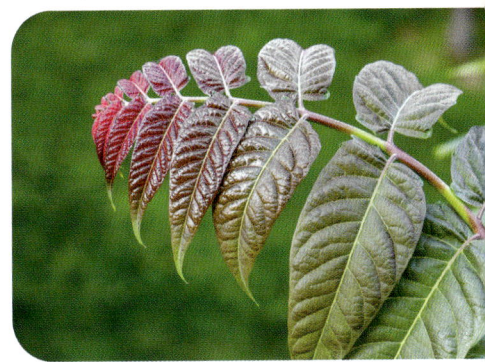

Sumac's new growth is reddish in color.

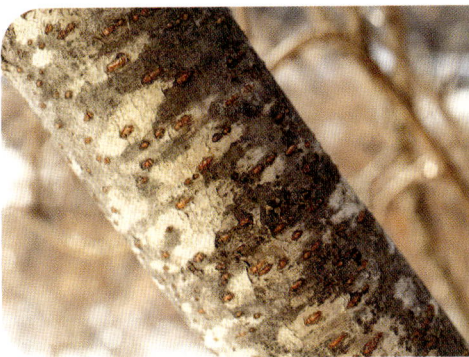

The mature bark of a sumac will have a pattern of dots or dashes (lenticels) on the surface.

BENEFITS

Nutritive. Rich in vitamins and minerals

Diuretic. Helps the body eliminate excess water through increased urination

Antibacterial. Inhibits bacterial growth

Astringent. Tonifies skin and smooth muscle tissue

IDENTIFICATION

Sumac trees can grow anywhere from 3 to 20 feet tall. They tend to grow in groups, with the mature bark developing lenticels (small pores that appear like dots or dashes on the bark), similar to elderberry. Younger bushes and

Avoiding Poison Sumac

To distinguish poison sumac from edible sumac, look for drooping white berries (instead of the upright red berries of edible sumac) and smooth twigs (instead of edible sumac's hairy ones).

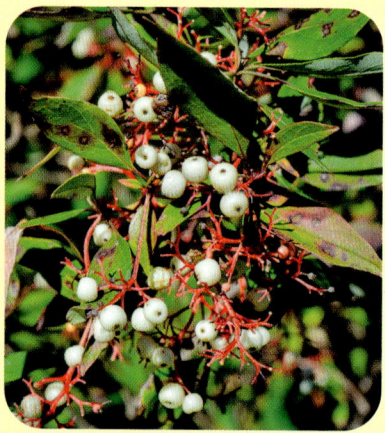

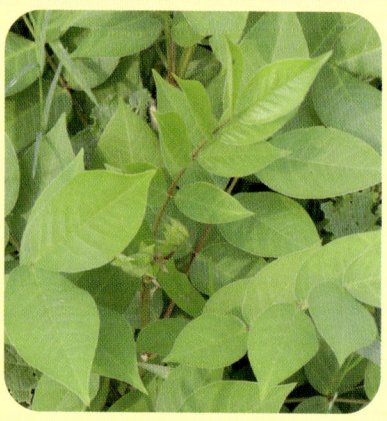

older plants with new growth will have fuzzy stems that turn reddish at the leaflets. Sumac's leaves are pinnately compound, with anywhere from 9 to 30 leaflets. The green leaves are darker on top than they are underneath and turn reddish orange in fall. The red fruits are covered in small, fine hairs and grow in clusters that point upward.

If you're worried about confusing sumac with poison sumac (*Toxicodendron vernix*), which can give you a rash like poison ivy, don't be; it's easy to tell them apart. The fruit clusters of edible sumac are red and point upward, whereas the fruit of poison sumac droops downward and matures to a whiteish color. Edible sumac's twigs are hairy, whereas poison sumac's are smooth. Finally, poison sumac loves to grow in swampy, moist areas. Edible sumac often grows along roadsides and in rocky soils and dry areas, all places that poison sumac avoids.

TRADITIONAL USAGE

Sumac, like many other plants native to the Americas, has an extensive history of being used for more than just medicine, especially by Indigenous peoples. This plant is used for tanning leather, dyeing fiber, making glue, and even making ink.

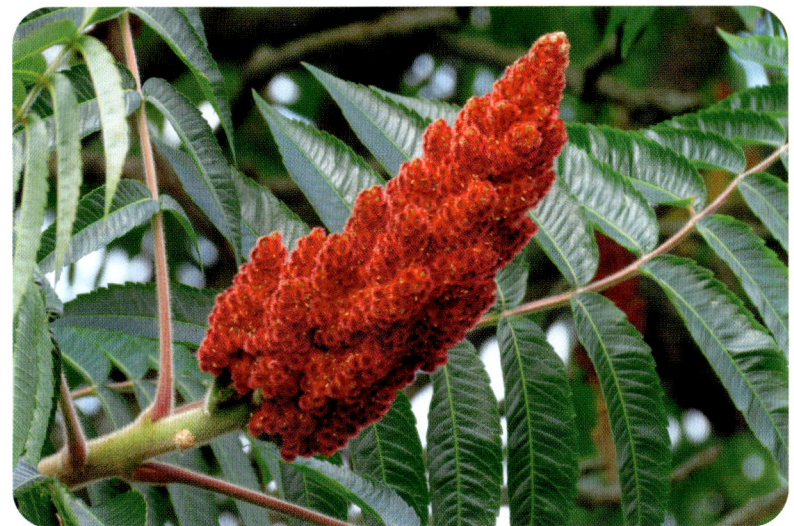

Sumac fruit can remain on the plant well into winter, but it's best to harvest it earlier in the season before it's damaged.

Aside from these uses, the berries and leaves are medicinal. The fruits, which are rich in tannins, can be boiled and drunk to ease digestive upset, diarrhea, urinary tract disorders, and cold and flu symptoms. They are also used for menstrual cramps and irregular menstruation. In the southern United States in more recent years, some communities use sumac as a medicine for sore throat, boiling both the leaves and fruits together for this purpose. The fruits are commonly picked fresh and made into sumac "lemonade," a tangy, delicious drink usually sweetened with honey or sugar (see page 243).

HARVESTING

Late summer to early fall is the best time of year to harvest sumac berries, though they can last on the plant for many months into winter. Some like to wait until the first frost to gather the berries, but later in the season I find they've been weathered and have lost much of their medicinal value. Bring pruners and cut the base of the fruit cluster, keeping it in a separate bag so the fruit isn't crushed in transit. Gather the foliage once the plant begins to leaf out in early summer, before the fruits are well developed.

PREPARATION

It can be difficult to separate sumac fruit from the stems. Try cutting each individual bunch off the main cluster, rolling your fingers over them until they separate. The seed itself is not used; it's the berry around the seed that holds the flavor and medicinal quality. If you want to powder sumac or use the pulverized berry in a blend, you can easily separate the two in a mortar and pestle or by crushing it with your hands. I prefer to do this after drying, as fresh berries can be a bit harder to remove without getting red juice all over your hands. You can leave the clusters whole for use in decoctions and teas.

Sumac berries are fairly dry, but it's best to give them some additional time to air-dry or put them in the dehydrator to ensure they don't mold. Fresh berries are great for making lemonade or any other drink, but especially ferments because the berries are covered in wild yeast. Once dried, they provide a strong citrusy taste and can be used for seasonings, marinades, and more. In many parts of the world, sumac shows up in spice blends such as za'atar and dukkha.

Although scurvy is no longer common, we can all use a good dose of vitamin C in winter, and sumac berries provide support for immunity and overall well-being. You can make sumac tea from the ripe berries as a nutritive, refreshing health boost. Sumac leaves can be harvested and used fresh to make a decoction, or dried and preserved for later use.

SUMAC FAST FACTS

- **Fruit clusters are vibrantly red, fuzzy, and point upward—unlike the drooping white fruit clusters of poison sumac**
- **Can grow anywhere from 3 to 20 feet tall**
- **Pinnately compound leaves with 9 to 30 leaflets**
- **New stem growth is hairy**
- **Tends to grow on forest edges and in rocky or dry soils, unlike poison sumac, which likes wet areas**
- **Leaves can be harvested throughout year, but especially in spring; harvest fruit clusters in fall and throughout winter as long as they remain vibrant red**

MIMOSA

Albizia julibrissin
Family: Fabaceae

Other Names: Persian silk tree

Parts Used: blossoms and bark

When to Harvest: spring, summer, and fall

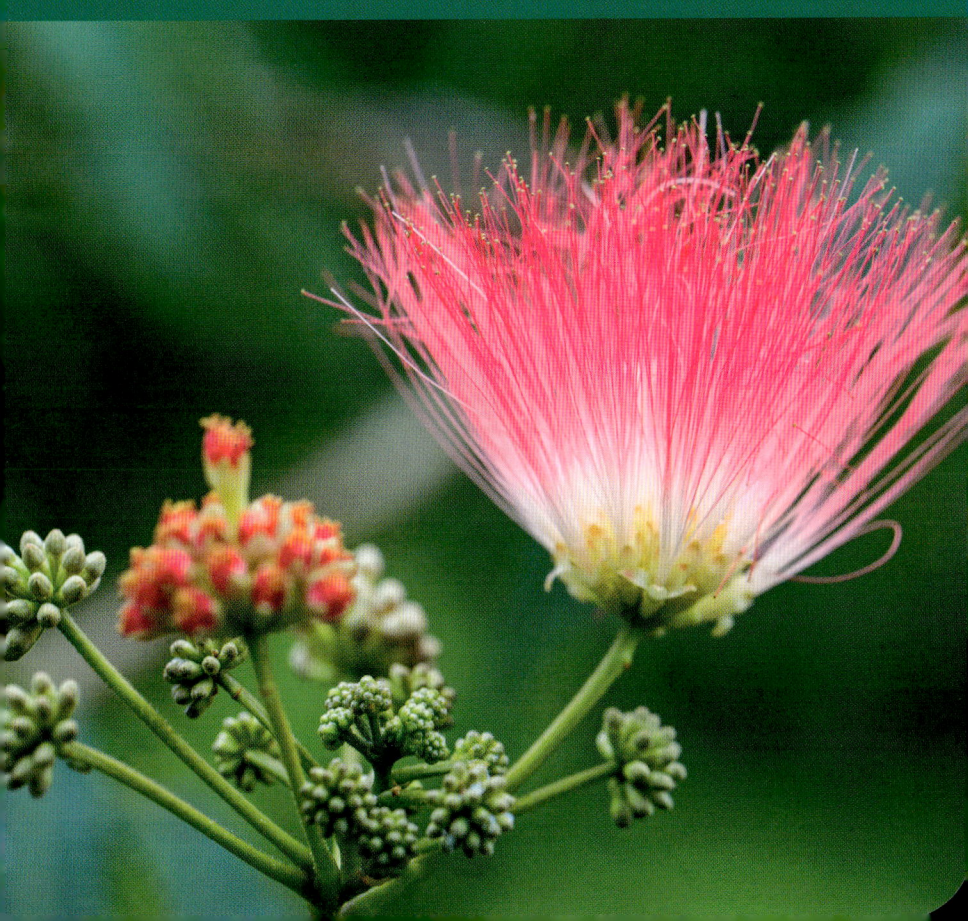

As summer blooms in the American South, so do the mimosa trees. In a season defined by vivid green, mimosa flowers are prolific enough to paint the landscape a bright shade of pink. Considered invasive in North America, this tree produces abundant seedpods and spreads very fast. It's known in the herbal community as a powerful plant ally, specifically for mental well-being.

BENEFITS

Nervine. Supports the nervous system

Anxiolytic. Eases anxiety

IDENTIFICATION

Mimosa trees grow up to 20 feet tall in temperate climates. The green leaves are alternate bi-pinnately compound (multiple pinnate leaves growing off a central stem), with clusters of flower buds at the end of the branches. The flowers are vibrantly pink with white at the base of the flower bud. The petals are erect, like tiny fireworks of color. The flowers will die back, leaving flat seedpods that dry out by fall. The tree's bark is a smooth brown-gray color. Mimosa trees can be found in disturbed

Mimosa trees thrive in disturbed areas. These fast-growing trees are often also used in landscaping.

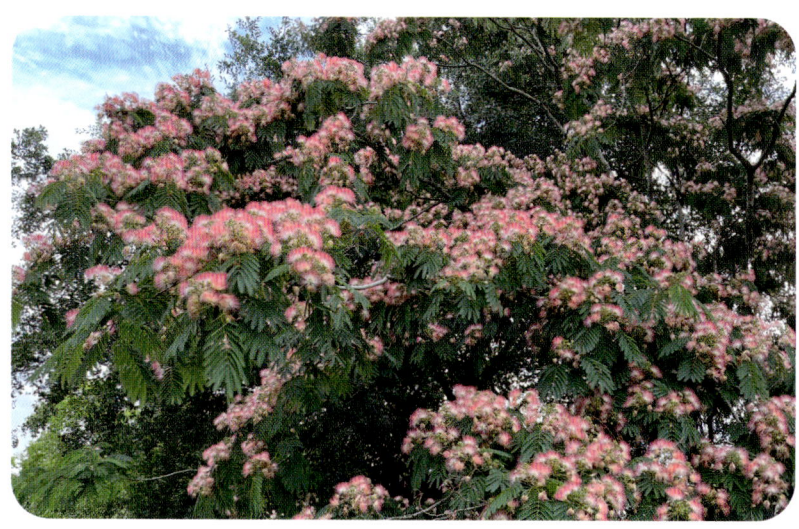

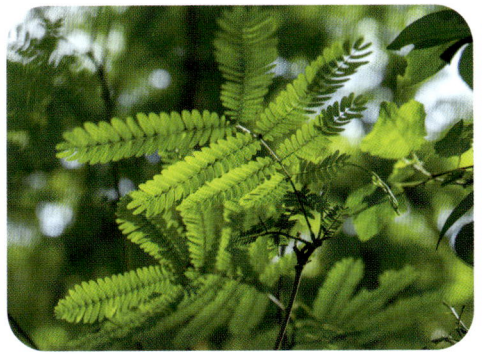
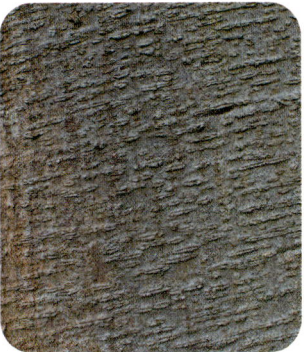

Mimosa leaves are bipinnately compound, with a feathery appearance. The bark is relatively smooth.

areas, landscaped into neighborhoods, or on forest edges, especially near construction.

TRADITIONAL USAGE

Native throughout Asia, this tree's bark, flowers, and stems are used in TCM as well as in herbal medical practices in Iran and Japan. Mimosa was introduced to North America in the 1700s and is now considered invasive. Typically, the flowers and bark are used medicinally; both have similar effects, but the flowers' tend to be milder. Calming and aromatic, mimosa flowers are a gentle nervine herb to ease anxiety and stress. Fresh flowers are more aromatic, but they can also be dried. The bark tends to work similarly and is boiled or tinctured to soothe the nervous system. In TCM, mimosa is specifically used to relieve suppressed emotions that may be detrimental to the body and mind.

HARVESTING

Harvest the blooming flowers in the middle of summer, simply plucking the flowers and stems off the branch. You can use them fresh the same day or dry them. Wait until late fall, after the blooms and seedpods are dried and falling off, to harvest the outer bark from the branches. The bark can also be harvested in spring, before the flowers appear.

Mimosa tends to be heavily branched, and harvesting the bark can be a good way to manage this fast-growing tree. Cut a large branch; then, using a sharp knife, carefully make a cut all the way down the branch, around its circumference and back up, creating two vertical lines on

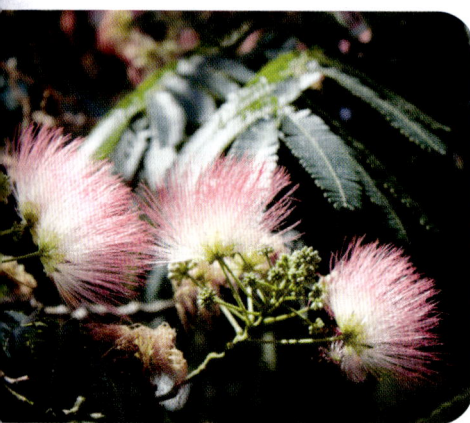

Mimosa flowers can be used fresh, the same day, or dried for later use.

MIMOSA FAST FACTS

- Bright pink blooms; white at base and turning pink at ends of petals
- Very small leaves; alternate, bi-pinnately compound
- Brownish gray, smooth bark
- Trees tend to grow on roadsides and in disturbed areas, not actually within forests
- Flowers are best harvested shortly after opening in summer; bark should be harvested in spring or fall after seedpods dry out
- Considered invasive; pick flowers so no seeds develop

opposite sides of the branch. Work the knife under the bark to slowly remove it. Always cut away from your body to prevent injury. The bark can be dried for use throughout winter.

PREPARATION

One of the most powerful medicinal aspects of mimosa is the calming aroma of the flowers. To take advantage of the lovely scent, make tea with the fresh or dried flowers, a vegetable glycerin extract with the fresh flowers, or even an infused floral honey! All of these preparations absorb the aroma and flavor well and capture the soothing qualities of the flowers. When using the bark, a decoction or tincture in high-proof alcohol are both ideal. If you wish to tincture the flowers, select a lower-proof alcohol to preserve the aromatic qualities. All of these preparations will support emotional well-being throughout the growing season and into winter.

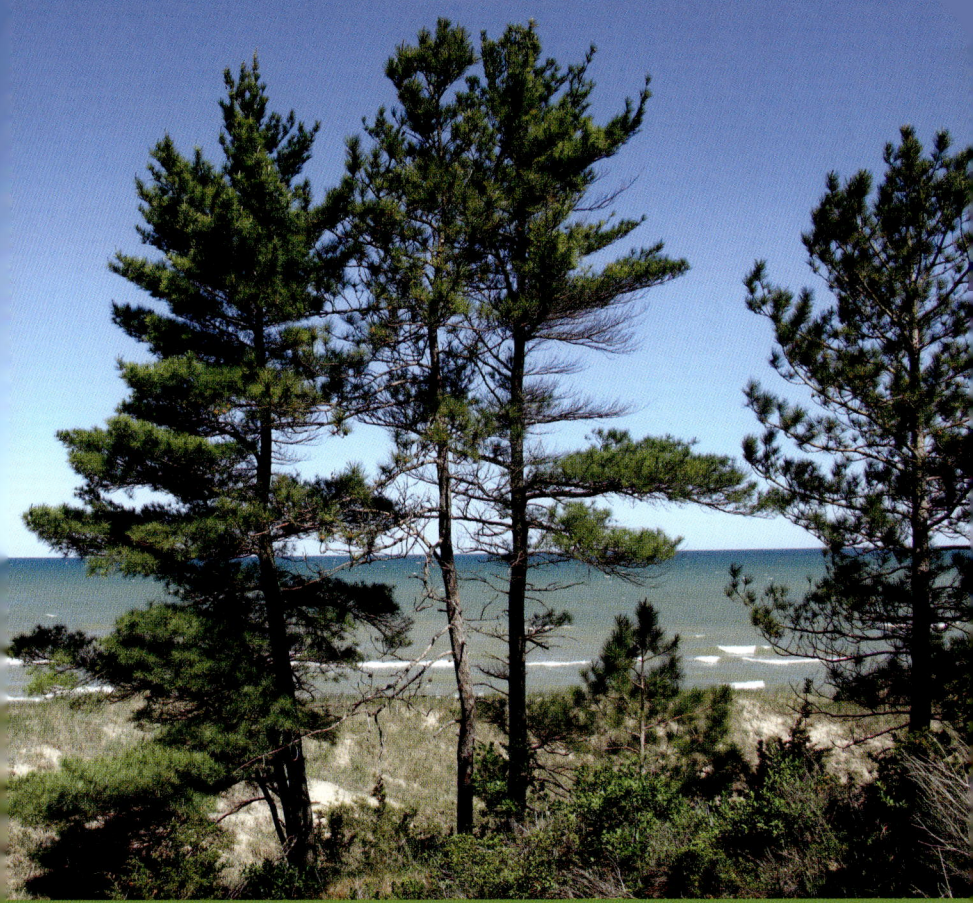

PINE

Pinus spp.
Family: Pinaceae

Parts Used: leaf tips, branch bark, unripe cones, and resin

When to Harvest: all year

A common evergreen throughout most temperate climates, the pine tree is an iconic part of landscapes across North America. Covered in vibrantly green needles, the entire tree can be used, from the pinecones and bark to the resin. Pines have been a staple source of medicine for Indigenous peoples throughout North America. Pine's aromatic quality is one of its best features; the smell conjures visions of being warm and cozy by the fire on a cold winter day.

BENEFITS

Analgesic. Pain reliever

Decongestant. Reduces nasal congestion

Warming carminative. Enhances digestion

Circulatory stimulant. Encourages blood flow

IDENTIFICATION

Pines are coniferous, evergreen trees that can grow up to 250 feet tall in some places. They grow throughout most of the temperate world. The bark is very distinct, becoming thick and scaly as the tree grows larger. Small

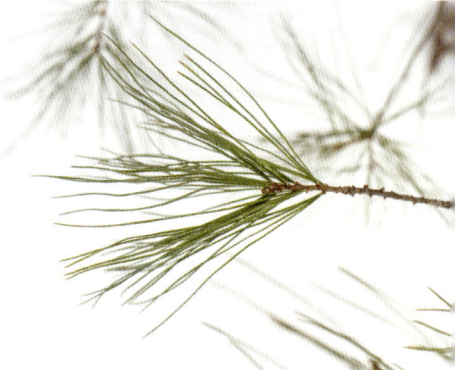

Pine needles grow in clumps of three to five.

layers can be peeled off the larger pieces once the tree is mature. Injured trees will commonly have a trail of resin dripping down from the point where the tree was damaged. Pine trees have needles that emerge in clusters of three to five, depending on the variety. These clusters distinguish pines from other needle-bearing trees such as spruce or fir. Pines produce cones at the end of mature branches, usually found higher up on the tree. The tree branches are whorled around the top of the trunk, usually dying on the lower sections as the tree grows taller. If you're ever in doubt, simply crushing the needles will release a distinct pine aroma.

TRADITIONAL USAGE

As an aromatic medicine, pine has been used extensively throughout the world.

The entire tree is used medicinally, sometimes even ceremonially. Pine's aromatic oils help increase circulation in the body. Pine baths and teas can be used to relieve body aches, headaches, swelling, and general pain. In baths and washes, pine can also be used to help relieve skin conditions such as psoriasis and eczema. Internally, pine needle tea can be taken for digestive upset, stomach infections, easing fever and cold symptoms, and coldness in the body.

Pine resin, which is found in all parts of the tree, is high in many essential oils, including *pinene*, a strongly aromatic oil that is powerfully analgesic, antimicrobial, and antifungal. It can be used for respiratory conditions such as cough and infection, chewed to cleanse the gums and for oral health, and for digestive upset. The resin is traditionally chewed, boiled, or tinctured in alcohol to release its medicinal qualities.

HARVESTING

Small pine branches often break during storms, making it easy to harvest the branches from the ground. Since the lower branches of pine trees tend to die off as the trees grow taller, using windfall branches is also much easier logistically—no need to climb 20 feet up! If you find a branch on the ground, use the needles, bark, and any unripe, aromatic

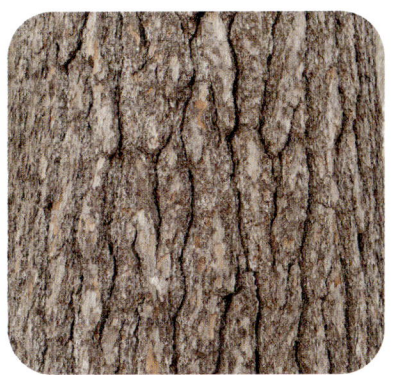

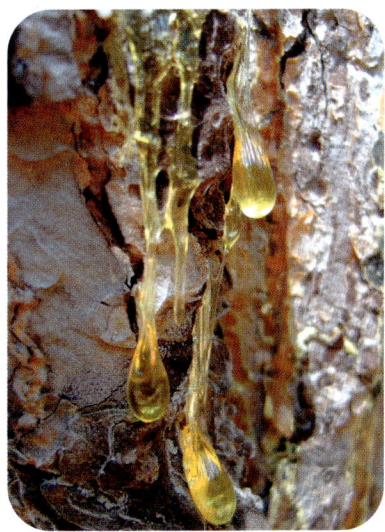

When gathering resin, don't break off resin oozing from a damaged area in the pine's bark, as that can further harm the tree. Instead look for drops of resin that have fallen on the trunk or on the forest floor.

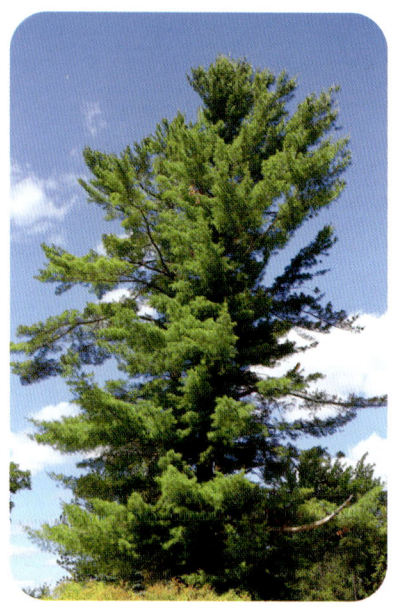

cones as well. The unripe cones are medicinal. Certain species of pine, like *Pinus contorta* and *P. rigida*, produce cones that, even if dried, contain resin that still retains medicinal benefits.

When gathering pine resin (or any resin), don't strip off resin from where it has seeped out from a cut or gash in the tree's bark. This is the tree's defense mechanism, and removing it will leave the tree vulnerable to infection. Instead, look on the forest floor below the resinous area to find "tears"—drops of resin that have fallen off the tree. If the resin is protruding extensively, breaking off a small piece without exposing the original wound is also a good approach.

PINE FAST FACTS

- Bark is distinctly textured with deep ridges
- Leaves are needles, emit pine aroma when crushed
- Needles grow in clusters of three to five
- Evergreen tree that can be harvested from year-round
- Tree branches whorl around tree
- All parts can be used, though tree bark tends to have less aromatic quality

PREPARATION

Combine fresh or dried pine needles to make an oil that will help with muscle soreness and circulation or that can be used as a general warming oil. Pine needles can be made into decoctions, vinegars, tinctures, and honeys to infuse their vibrant aroma and aromatic qualities. A tincture made from the resin is great for a cold, as a mouthwash, for sinus congestion, and more.

REISHI

Ganoderma tsugae, Ganoderma lucidum
Family: Ganodermataceae

Other Names: ling zhi

Parts Used: fruiting body of the fungus

When to Harvest: spring

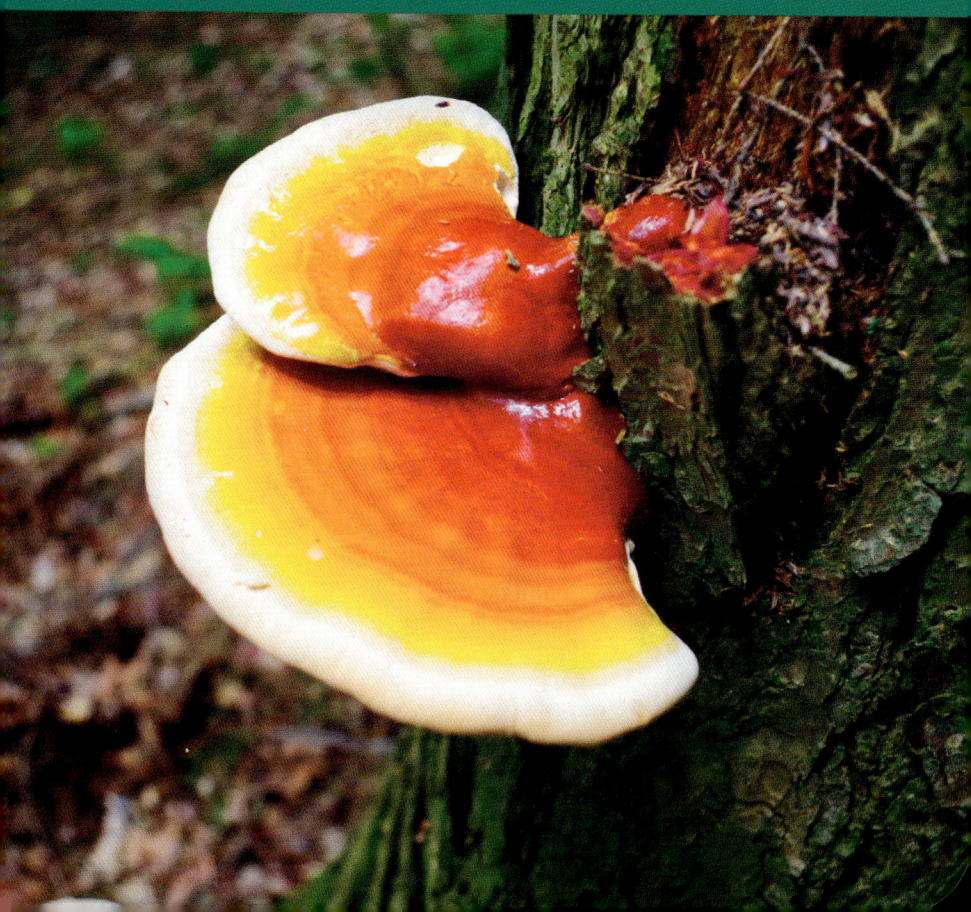

A staple in TCM and now used throughout the Western world, reishi mushroom can be found in just about every form: powders, capsules, tinctures, and whole. Reishi is a common fungus. The most frequently used species (*Ganoderma tsugae*) tends to grow in hemlock forests on the East Coast or on other hardwoods throughout the Americas. You might also spot *G. lucidum*, another species that is native to Asia but commonly cultivated, on dead tree stumps. Reishi is a powerful aid to the immune system and nourishes the cardiovascular system—both effects that just about everyone could benefit from. Considering the stress, environmental issues, overwork, and general chaos of modern-day life, we could all use some support, and reishi is a perfect way to get it.

BENEFITS

Cardiovascular tonic. Supports the cardiovascular system

Immunomodulator. Modulates the immune system

Antiviral. Supports the body in combating viruses

Look for reishi mushrooms with a white edge of new growth, which indicates they are fresh and tender.

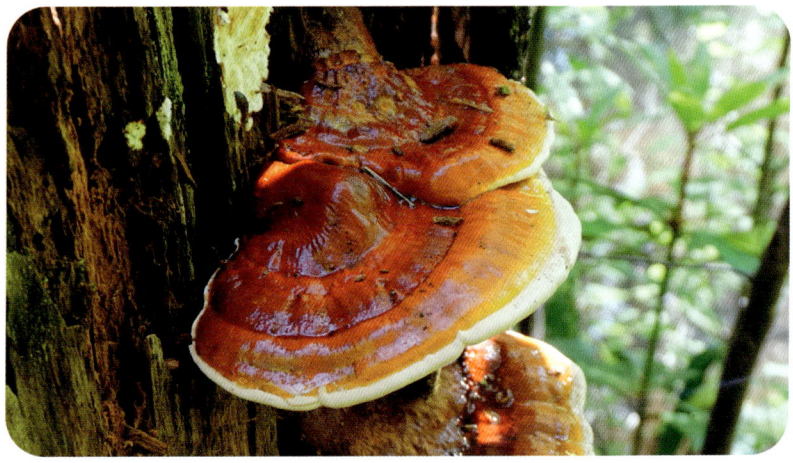

IDENTIFICATION

The reishi mushroom is a polypore, meaning it does not grow up from the ground with a stem and cap but rather grows directly off its host, usually a log or dying tree. Polypores are also identified by their pores, or small dots on the bottom side of the mushroom, which release spores for future propagation. When it first emerges, reishi is a vibrant red, often with a band of white at the tender outermost edge. In its prime you may see still some tender, white edges, but most of the mushroom will be vivid shades of deep red and orange. The surface of the mushroom has a distinctly shiny, varnished look that makes it easy to identify.

Reishi likes to grow on hardwoods, either dead or alive, particularly on eastern hemlock trees. Some species, such as G. lucidum, grow on dead wood. They may appear to be growing directly from the ground but are actually attached to dead root systems beneath the soil. You may notice brownish red spores coating the top of the mushroom or releasing from the underside when tapped. Reishi mushrooms vary in size, from a few inches to almost a foot and a half in length.

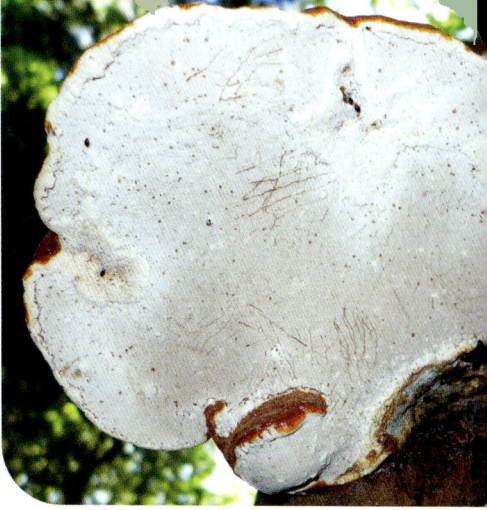

Polypore mushrooms, like reishi, have visible pores on the underside.

TRADITIONAL USAGE

Reishi has been used globally and has a reputation in TCM for being a powerful tonic for longevity and wellness. It contains a myriad of medicinal compounds that affect the cardiovascular system and nourish the lungs and heart, helping facilitate blood flow and healthy circulation. Reishi's bitter flavor is due to the presence of *triterpenoids*, medicinal compounds that nourish the gut and stimulate digestion, regulate inflammation and immune activity, and are even active against viral infections. It's considered a medicine for both the nervous system and the spirit, helping regulate sleep cycles, calm the mind, and buffer the body during times of stress.

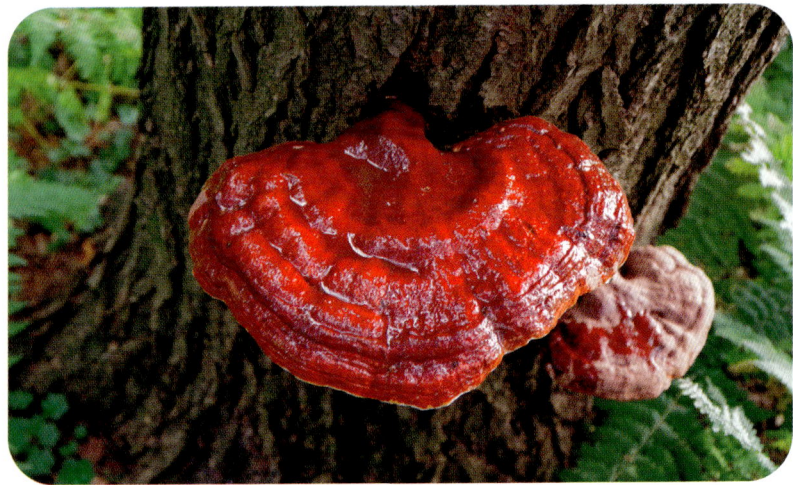

Reishi can vary in color from deep red to a rich orange or brown.

Reishi is an *adaptogen*. An adaptogen is an herb or substance that has a unique regulating effect on the body, depending on the situation. For instance, in the evening, a cup of reishi tea will help ease the body into sleep. In the morning, however, the same tea will help kick-start processes in the body and wake up the system, getting you ready for your day. Similarly, if taken when the immune system isn't functioning well, it will stimulate activity. Taken when the immune system is overstimulated, it will lower and modulate immune activity. Adaptogens help bring our bodies into equilibrium and balance. Reishi is a powerful adaptogen, which is why I take some of my reishi mushroom tincture every day, no matter the scenario!

HARVESTING

When harvesting reishi, be mindful of how many are growing in the area, as you would with any plant. While reishi is abundant, it's also vital to the environment, often serving as a home and food source for many other creatures (check out the underside of a reishi mushroom past its harvestable prime and you'll see a host of insects). Like other fungi, it plays an essential role in breaking down organic material and replenishing the soil and earth.

Bring a sharp knife or pruners when you harvest, and cut the part of the mushroom closest to the tree, being careful not to rip it off and damage the bark. Various species of reishi can grow year-round, but G. *tsugae* and G. *lucidum* like to grow in the moist spring rains, especially in hardwood forests. I've spent many years exploring the forests of western North Carolina, and in the months of April and May I have often come across lush green forests dotted with the vibrant reds of reishi.

A good reishi mushroom will be firm, glossy on top, and slightly moist, with a nice cream-white color on the bottom. Once you process it, you'll see how much medicine a few of these can make!

PROCESSING

Reishi mushroom is best used dry, as the fresh fungus has a high water content that dilutes its usefulness. Make sure you're ready to process your harvest the same day, as this mushroom dries quickly. Once dry, cutting it will be like chopping an old log in half.

Cut your reishi with the grain, so to speak, from the point it was attached to the tree outward, in small, quarter-inch slices. Dry the slices in the sun or in a dehydrator until firm, making sure they are fully dried. If you want to make tea, break them down further by snapping the dried slices into three or four pieces and make a decoction, boiling your water and fungus together for 15 to 20 minutes. Reishi needs to be kept at a rolling boil long enough to extract its medicine. After boiling and steeping, the decoction will have a yellow-orange color. Reishi, like many medicinal mushrooms, is not edible raw!

REISHI FAST FACTS

- Polypore mushroom, growing directly off trees, with pores visible on underside
- Top of fungus is a vibrant red, orange, and yellow with a white band of new growth on outer edge and a shiny, varnished appearance
- Various species, some growing directly off dead stumps
- Best harvested in spring in moist forests
- Ranges in length from a few inches to a foot and a half
- This mushroom plays a vital role in forest ecosystems; be mindful of how much you harvest

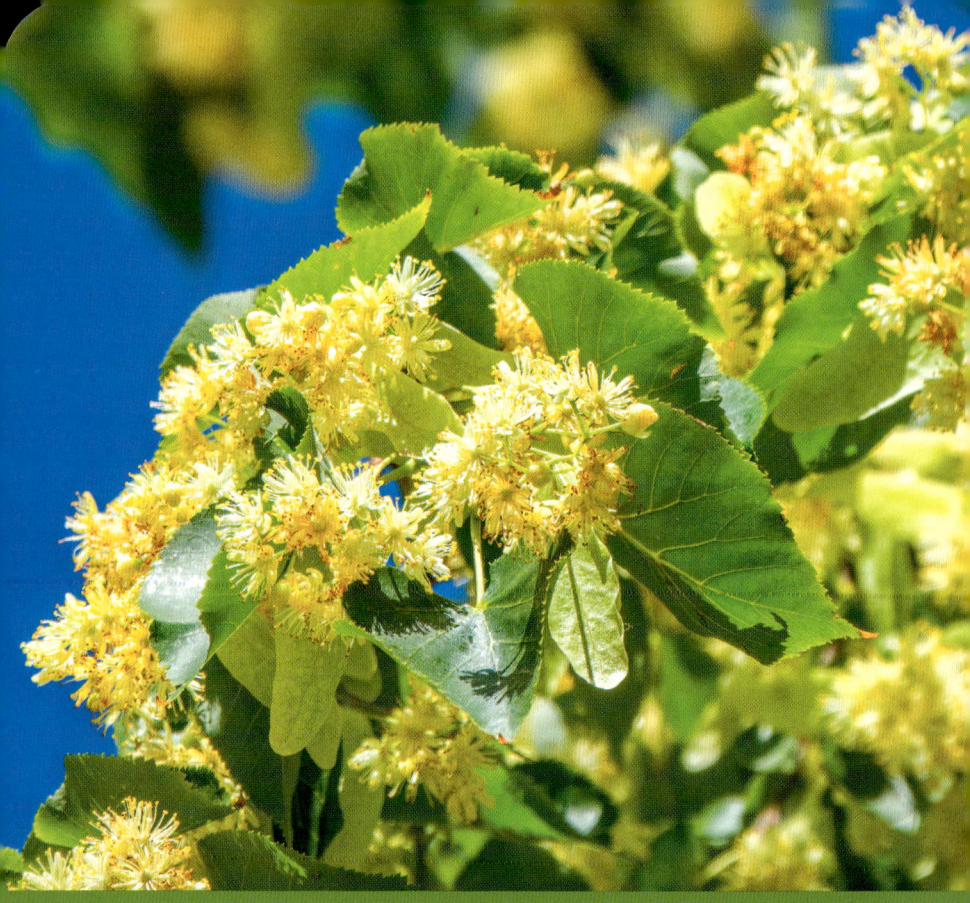

LINDEN

Tilia spp.
Family: Malvaceae

Other Names: basswood, tilia

Parts Used: blossoms

When to Harvest: summer

I associate the sweet scent of the linden tree with an unexpected place: New York City. I recall wandering through the city streets in early summer, smelling the linden flowers blooming on every street corner and hearing the eager buzzing of bees as they collected nectar from every blossom. Linden trees are often planted ornamentally along roadsides and in neighborhoods, hence their presence in New York. The aromatic blooms are used for medicine and help nourish our nervous systems, easing us into sleep in higher doses or simply keeping us calm throughout the day. Little tea bags of "tila" or "tilo," filled with linden flowers, are commonly found in Latin America and used medicinally in that region.

BENEFITS

Anxiolytic. Eases anxiety

Demulcent. Cooling and soothing

Diaphoretic. Increases sweating to break fever

The serrated leaves of the linden tree are dark green on the top and lighter on the underside.

IDENTIFICATION

Linden is a tree native to the Americas that can grow up to 100 feet tall. Its serrated leaves are dark green on top, with a lighter shade on the underside. The triangular heart shape of this leaf is distinct, and the abundant flowers make linden even easier to identify. The flowers emerge in clusters of white and yellow, emitting a powerfully floral aroma that is sure to stop you in your tracks. Depending on your location, you may see bees hovering around them, as they are a great source of nectar. The flowers emerge alongside a *subtending bract* that is unique to a linden. It looks like an elongated leaf, though a little smaller and lighter in color, that is attached at the base of the flower stems and hangs down alongside the blooms.

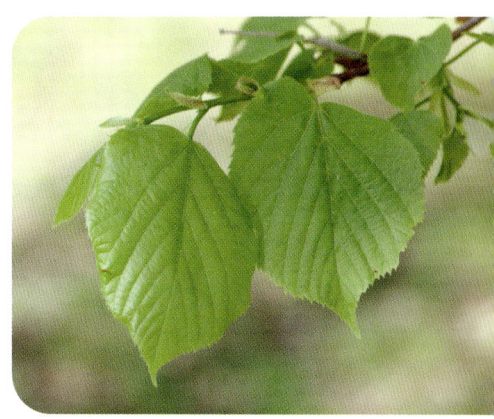

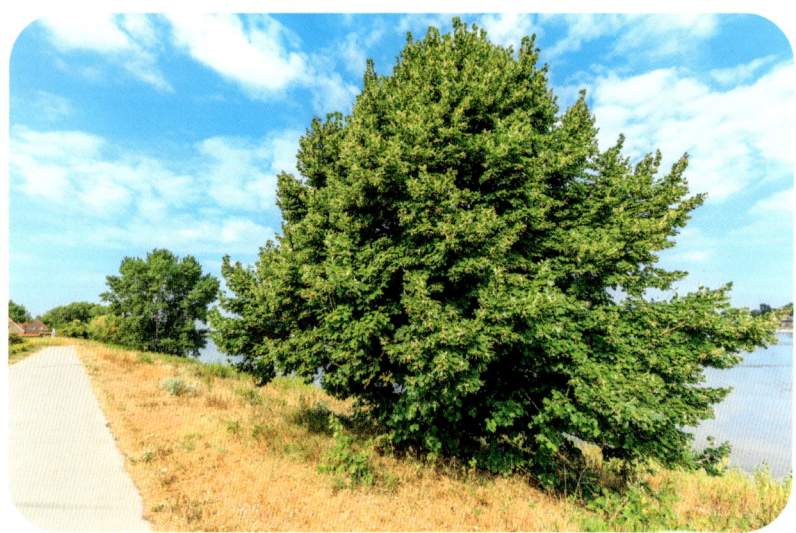

Linden is often planted ornamentally along roadsides.

TRADITIONAL USAGE

Linden flower is a common medicine used to nourish the nervous system. As an anxiolytic, it helps ease anxiety, quieting the mind and supporting sleep. It can also be helpful during the day, easing tension and stress. Linden is great for people who feel they are running around with a million thoughts on their mind; it helps them avoid that frantic tendency during the day and put aside their stress at night. Much of linden's medicine is in its sweet, calming aroma. The chemical compound *tricosane* is one of many aromatic compounds in these flowers; it's the same compound found in magnolia flowers and even vanilla.

Linden is in the Malvaceae family, also known as the mallow family, and it is rich in mucilage (the same slimy substance that comes from okra when you chop it up raw). Mucilage is cooling and demulcent, coating the digestive tract and other parts of the system while soothing and nourishing these tissues. This makes linden ideal for digestive upset and mild respiratory ailments. As a diaphoretic, linden increases sweating. It is gentle but strong and is commonly combined with other aromatics to help lower fever and calm the body after sickness.

HARVESTING

Depending on where you are, linden will bloom in early to midsummer. The flowers are best harvested within a day or two of blooming, so keep an eye on your trees as the season approaches. The flowers will lose their aromatic qualities, one of their most medicinal aspects, within a few days of being open and even faster due to rain. A potent, floral aroma is a good indicator that the blooms are ready to harvest. Make sure that you use them the same day as harvesting or dry them quickly to preserve the aroma! You can harvest the flowers together with their bract, the small, ovular leaf attached. Use pruners and cut the flower stems where they connect to the tree to make sure you don't damage the branch.

PROCESSING

Once harvested, make tea with the fresh blossoms or put them in a dehydrator to preserve their aroma and medicine. You can also leave them on a tray in a spot with good airflow and they will dry within a few days. If using them fresh, the flowers are excellent in simple syrups or honey infusions, since the smell pairs well with sweet, sugary preparations. For the same reason, avoid alcohol when tincturing linden blossoms and instead use vegetable glycerin to complement the aroma with sweetness. Linden syrup or honey can be added to teas and substituted in recipes calling for a liquid sweetener to add a calming floral note.

LINDEN FAST FACTS

- Commonly planted in urban areas and in cities
- Triangular ovate leaves with serrated edges
- Leafy, ovular subtending bract attached to flowering parts
- Flowers bloom whiteish yellow and are strongly aromatic in summer
- Smooth, vertically ridged, gray-brown bark
- Flowers best harvested soon after opening, when they are most aromatic

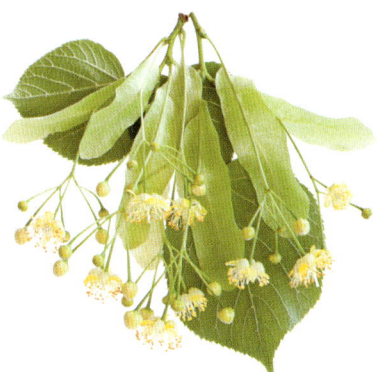

Linden blossoms have a subtending bract that looks like a smaller, lighter leaf growing alongside the blooms.

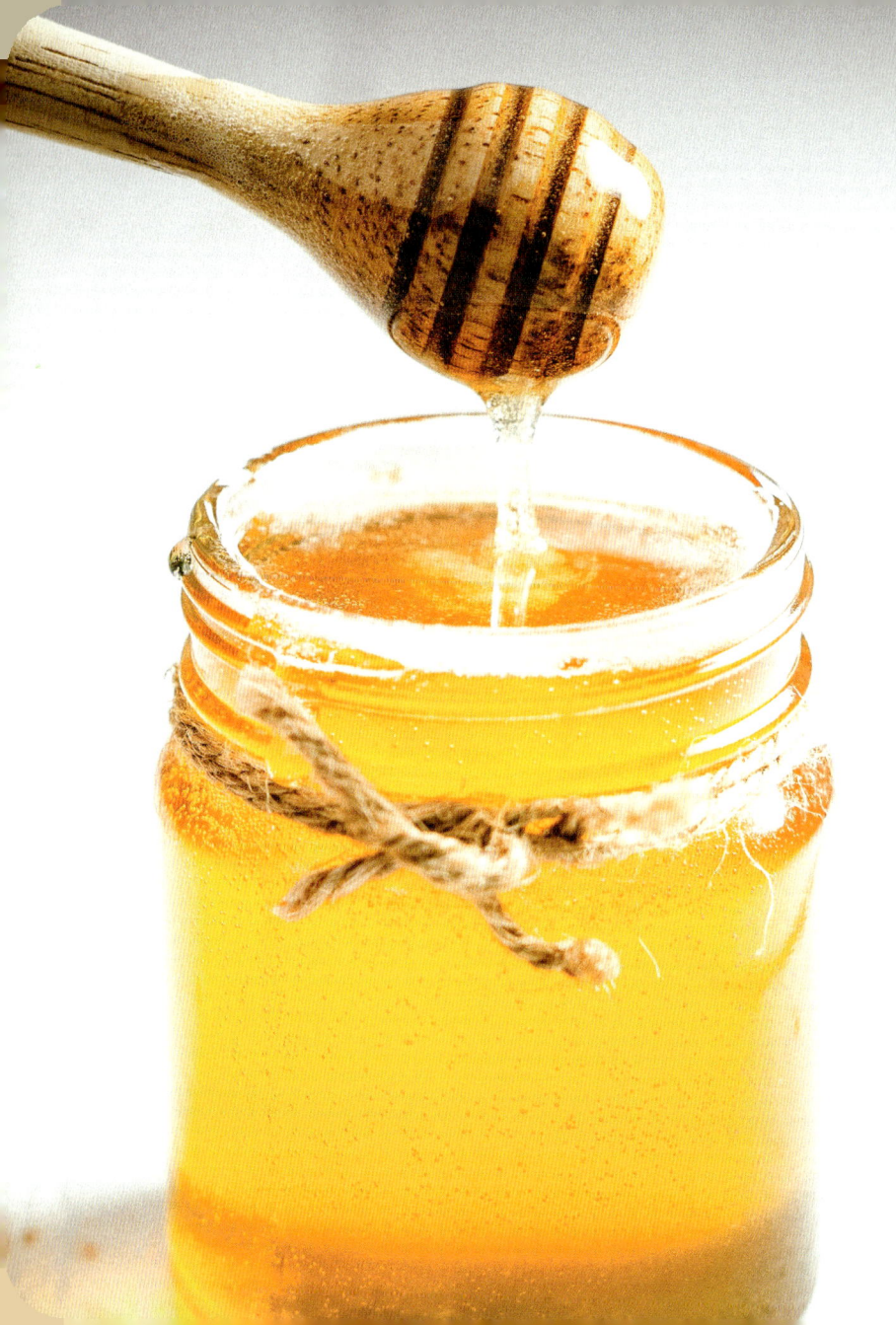

CHAPTER 7

Making MEDICINE

Our plant allies are full of powerful medicinal compounds that can soothe and nourish our bodies, which makes the journey from raw plant material to healing medicine surprisingly simple. You'll just need some basic supplies and tools to get started.

Understanding Plant Medicine

What exactly is plant medicine? I define plant medicine as any preparation of a plant that's designed to extract its healing qualities for therapeutic use. That often involves using a solution of alcohol, vinegar, or water to extract those qualities. Of course, you can benefit from the medicinal effects by simply eating many of these plants (more on that in the next chapter), but these healing properties can also be concentrated for acute applications.

While recipes are very useful (and you'll find several in the next chapter), I have developed many of my medicine-making techniques using my senses to gauge the potency, flavors extracted, and ratios. Making plant medicine is an art that is deeply intertwined with that of making food, and the same sense of instinct and curiosity needed to cook will serve you well in making medicine.

Making Medicine Safely

Plants are natural, but this does not mean they can't do us harm. Just as we want to be completely sure that we have positively identified a plant, there are also some basic precautions to take while making and consuming medicines.

All the plants in this book can be ingested generously without side effects, but it's important to remember that everybody is different, literally. Every body is different. I drink chamomile tea during the day to ease stress and focus better; meanwhile, a cup of chamomile tea would put my dad to sleep in the workplace. We all absorb compounds differently.

CONSIDER POSSIBLE DRUG INTERACTIONS. While plants are different in many ways from pharmaceuticals, herbal medicines may interact with medications you're taking. Never replace

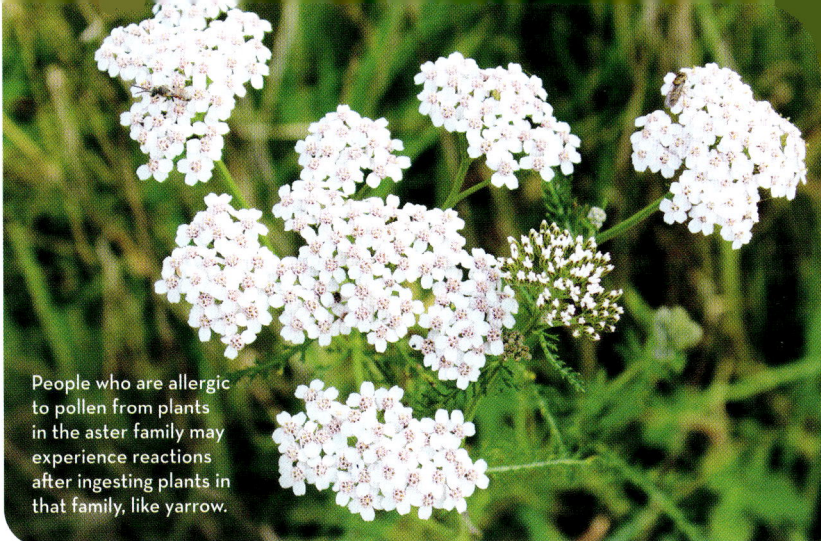

People who are allergic to pollen from plants in the aster family may experience reactions after ingesting plants in that family, like yarrow.

prescribed medications with herbal medicines without first consulting a professional. If you're currently on medication, always seek the guidance of a healthcare professional or trusted, accredited herbalist before adding herbal medicine to your routine. Listen to your body and to your general healthcare practitioner before and while taking herbal medicines. Conferring with a professional helps ensure you'll benefit fully from the medicinal qualities of our plant allies.

BE AWARE OF ALLERGENS. Before you ingest a new plant, it's important to be mindful of a possible immune system response. Take a small amount of a new preparation or plant and see if you notice any symptoms or reactions. Most times there will be no issue, but it's better to be cautious. For instance, some folks who are allergic or sensitive to the aster family may sneeze or have a runny nose after ingesting related plants in that family. Tune in to your body and keep this in mind when using any new plant, just like when trying a new food.

HERBAL MEDICINE AND PREGNANCY. There are usage warnings in Chapters 4 to 6 for all the plants profiled in this book that can have potentially negative side effects for certain populations. In particular, sweet Annie, mugwort, Japanese knotweed, wild lettuce, motherwort, and Oregon grape should all be avoided by people who are pregnant, nursing, or hoping to become pregnant. If you are pregnant or nursing, it's best to be particularly cautious about introducing herbal medicine to your diet; always consult with a healthcare provider.

DOSAGE. You'll find general dosage suggestions in the following pages, and in most cases there isn't a risk from taking "too much." However, in plant medicine *more* doesn't automatically mean *better*. You don't ever need to be drinking whole pints of tincture. The goal is to find a balance that works for your body. Start at a low dosage, observe how the medicine impacts you and adjust accordingly.

What You'll Need to Make Herbal Medicine

You likely already have many of the supplies and ingredients you'll need to make herbal medicines, but we'll explore some of the key items that can make things simple.

MENSTRUUM

In herbal terms, a *menstruum* is a liquid used for making medicine. Different menstrua extract different compounds, have different flavors, and offer different energetics. Let's talk about some of the basics: water, oil, vinegar, honey, alcohol, and vegetable glycerin.

WATER. The universal solvent, and the most common liquid to use for making medicine, is water. It can be used in teas, infusions, and decoctions. It's also the menstruum of choice for making washes, herbal rinses for the hair or body, and steams (where herbs are boiled, and the aromatic steam is inhaled for respiratory conditions). Make sure you're using clean water—whether that's spring water, filtered water, or tap water, depending on your local source.

OIL. Made up of fats, oil is used to extract fat-soluble compounds such as aromatic essential oils and other oils found in plants. The molecules in the menstruum oil bond with the oils naturally present in the plant, drawing them out. Oil is great for topical applications that can be rubbed into the body; herbal infused oils, such as garlic oil and rosemary oil, are also excellent for cooking. You can use a variety of neutral oils as a menstruum. Extra- virgin olive oil is the most common (usually called EVOO in the herbal world), along with grape-seed oil, avocado oil, sesame oil, and sunflower oil.

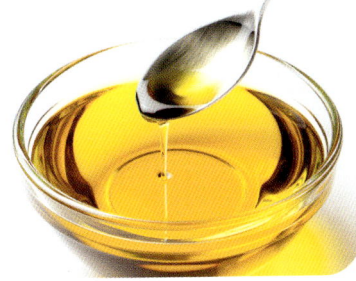

Extra-virgin olive oil is the one most commonly used in herbalism, but you can use whatever neutral oil you prefer.

VINEGAR. The acetic acid and water in vinegar, specifically apple cider vinegar, help extract flavors and aromatic compounds. Apple cider vinegar is very pungent and has a positive impact on the digestive system and respiratory tract, making it a good menstruum to use with plants that have an affinity for these parts of the body. Apple cider vinegar

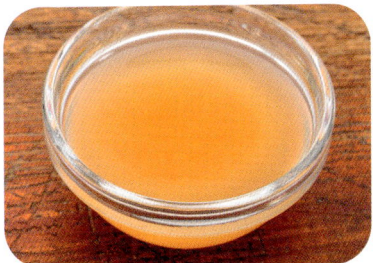

Apple cider vinegar offers health benefits of its own, even before being combined with medicinal plants, making it an excellent menstruum.

What You'll Need to Make Herbal Medicine

also extracts more vitamins and minerals than preparations like alcohol or oil, which is why it's a great menstruum to make a multivitamin vinegar using plants like stinging nettle.

HONEY. Honey is a more fragile menstruum and doesn't tolerate high heat. It efficiently captures aromatic oils and flavors but isn't a good choice for releasing compounds that need to be extracted by consistent boiling. I prefer to use local raw honey, if possible, as some "honey" bought at the store is actually partially sugar or glucose syrup. Honey can be medicinal for the respiratory system and is great for plants that are used for cough, cold, sore throat, and so forth. Some roots, such as ginger, can be chopped well and infused into honey, if they're minced finely enough to open the surface area and release the flavors and compounds.

ALCOHOL. Alcohol, specifically ethyl alcohol (ethanol), is the most-used menstruum for making tinctures, efficiently extracting medicinal compounds from plants, especially the tougher, more fibrous ones. Alcohol extracts the same components as water but in a more thorough manner. It also captures compounds such as alkaloids. (Alkaloids are secondary metabolites that work very efficiently and strongly on the body; nicotine is perhaps the most familiar, but there are many more.)

Higher-proof alcohol is better for roots and other fibrous materials. You can use vodka, tequila, or any liquor with an alcohol percentage of 20 to 50 for leaves and flowers, but choose rum, Everclear, and other higher-percentage alcohols (50 to 80 percent) for roots and barks. Technically, you can use any alcohol sold for humans to drink; I have a tasty Hennessy–holy basil tincture. Alcohol has a very hot, drying energy, so bear that in mind when considering the condition being addressed and long-term use.

The Difference Between Alcohol by Volume and Proof

Alcohol by volume (ABV) and proof are two ways of designating how much alcohol is in liquor. *ABV* refers to the percentage of alcohol content in a liquid. The *proof* is equal to double the ABV of a given liquor. So a 90-proof whiskey is 45 percent alcohol by volume. This book uses ABV, but you will also commonly see liquor labeled by proof.

VEGETABLE GLYCERIN. Vegetable glycerin is a thick, viscous liquid made from plant oils. Glycerin is sweet and acts as an extractive liquid. It's a great option for those who don't consume alcohol and for children who dislike the flavor of alcohol in tinctures. However, it's not as strong an extractive as alcohol. Use it for well-crushed roots along with leaves or flowers. I prefer glycerin derived from coconut, because others can be made from either palm or soy from questionable sources. Be sure to purchase culinary-grade vegetable glycerin, as it is also sold for topical use.

HELPFUL TOOLS

Many of the tools you'll need to make medicine are common kitchen items, but there are some specialty tools that will be useful.

POTS. You'll be boiling water, steaming plants, and boiling jars in various pots, so it's ideal to have several. Having a range of sizes will allow you to choose how large a batch of medicine you wish to make. Be sure your pot has a tight-fitting lid, as the preparation often needs to be covered while it steeps or boils.

STRAINER OR PRESS. Strainers are useful for removing fine particles from your preparation before consuming. Bits of remaining plants can affect the texture of salves and oils and can lead to mold or spoilage. Even if you're making a basic infusion or decoction, having bits of root or leaf caught in your throat isn't ideal.

I keep both fine-mesh strainers and strainers with larger holes on hand. Ball strainers are useful for making infusions; they're small mesh spheres that can be filled with herbs before pouring boiling water over them. I prefer stainless steel strainers; be mindful of plastic versions, as heat can pull out chemicals that you don't want to consume.

A handheld tincture press is especially helpful when pressing tinctures, oils, or anything you want to fully extract liquids from. They can be bought online and have a squeezing mechanism and a strainer at the bottom, allowing you to force all the liquid from your preparation without dropping bits and pieces into your final product.

MASON JARS. These heat-safe jars are the perfect container for making and storing tinctures. They can be bought in packs of 12 or in bulk online or in most supermarkets. They come in various sizes, from 4 ounces all the way up to 64 ounces. Since they are made of glass, you don't need to worry about the toxic chemicals that can be found in some plastics. Mason jars are made of tempered glass, but always be cautious when rapidly heating or cooling glass to prevent cracking.

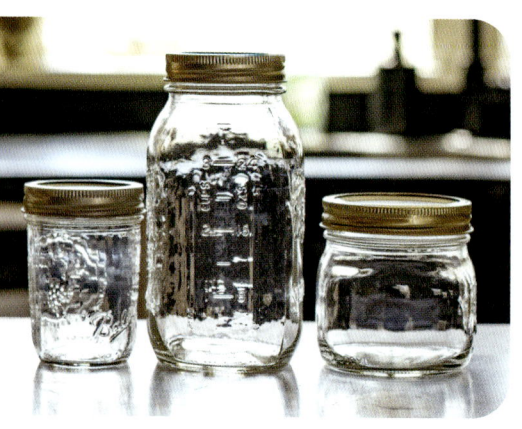

FUNNEL. A funnel is helpful to prevent spills when you're filling a jar. Look for an option that's heat-safe.

DROPPER BOTTLES. These are great for bottling finished medicine and administering it. The built-in dropper allows you to accurately measure out the correct dosage. Amber bottles are best, as they protect the contents from sunlight, which might degrade the medicine. I prefer one- to two-ounce bottles, but I use larger bottles for medicines taken daily.

KITCHEN SCALE. A scale allows you to accurately measure the weight of your ingredients when making medicines.

MIXING BOWLS. I find it easier to strain tinctures into a mixing bowl before portioning them into smaller dropper bottles, rather than straining directly into the bottles. Ceramic, glass, or metal are often better choices than plastic.

SCISSORS OR KNIFE. These can be used to chop up plant materials such as stems and leaves.

LABELS. Always label your medicine the day you make it. Labeling is important; otherwise you'll quickly find yourself mixing up medicines or unsure of what a bottle contains. Some people make intricate labels that have space to write where something was harvested, the ratio used, if it was fresh or dry, and other details. That information can be helpful to record, but a simple label that indicates the contents of the jar and the date is sufficient ("Stinging Nettle in Vodka 03/20/26").

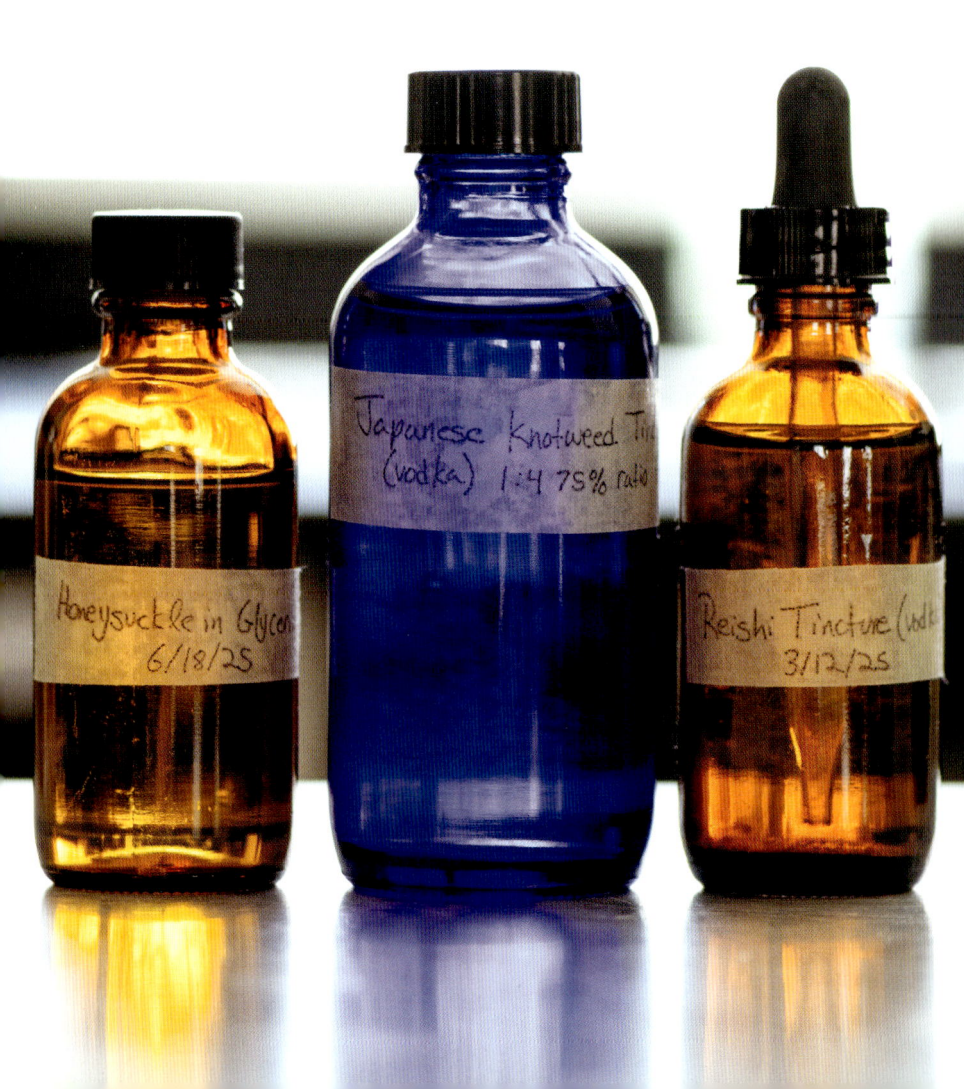

CHAPTER 8

Base Recipes FOR MAKING MEDICINE

The base recipes in this chapter offer a blueprint for making medicines, with guidelines on how much herb to use, simple step-by-step directions, suggestions on how to store the finished medicine, and dosage recommendations.

NOW THAT YOU'VE GATHERED YOUR SUPPLIES, let's look at some recipes! Each of these base recipes can be adapted to various plants, depending on what you have available and what type of medicine you wish to make. After each base recipe, you'll find suggested plants that could benefit from that specific approach. However, don't be afraid to experiment, mixing and matching various preparations with different plants. The suggested plants are just the beginning! The more you experiment and explore, the more you'll learn about these plants and how to use them.

Infusions

An herbal infusion is made by bringing water to a boil, pouring it over fresh or dried herbs, and allowing them to steep to extract their therapeutic compounds. For many people, this is the most common method of working with herbs. The process of making an infusion is essentially the same as making tea, so you've likely already made one if you've brewed yourself a cup of chamomile or mint tea.

MAKING A STRONG INFUSION

When making an infusion, the water is poured directly onto the herbs, so the temperature drops rapidly instead of being sustained for a longer period. This means that only certain compounds will be extracted, and herbal infusions may not be as potent as other preparations. Infusions are best made with plant materials that are well broken down, whether fresh or dry, particularly leaves, flowers, and stems. More fibrous plant material, such as roots, seeds, and bark, often need consistent boiling, through decoction, to extract their medicines.

The longer an infusion steeps the more medicinal compounds will be extracted—up to a certain point. For example, most black tea is steeped for a few minutes. If you leave it for 10 minutes, it will

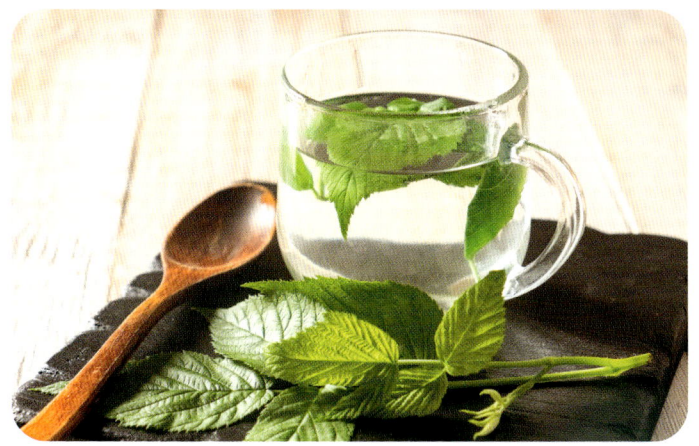

become overly astringent or bitter. That's because the tannins in the tea leaves continue to be extracted by the residual heat. An oversteeped cup of tea might not be ideal, but in the case of making plant medicine, a more potent mixture can be helpful. Many herbs release even more of their medicinal qualities when steeped overnight, but an infusion will usually reach its maximum extraction within 24 hours. So, no, unfortunately your infusion will not be the most powerful if you left it to steep for a week; it probably extracted to its fullest extent 5 days ago.

Infusion, Tea, or Decoction?

Throughout this book, the term *infusion* is used to refer to a medicine made by pouring boiling water over herbs and letting them steep. *Tea* is a more general term that describes water-based medicines including infusions as well as *decoctions*, which are made by bringing water and plant material to a rolling boil for a longer period of time.

MAKING AND STORING AN INFUSION

Always make sure to cover your infusions after pouring them, allowing them to cool to a drinkable temperature while covered. This keeps the volatile oils and medicinal compounds from escaping in steam.

At room temperature, infusions will last a day or two, possibly less, depending on the plant used (especially if it's a fruit or very water-dense plant). In the refrigerator, an infusion can last about a week. A general rule of thumb is to use one to two tablespoons of dried herb per cup of water for this preparation. With fresh herbs, double this amount to two to four tablespoons, as the plant material still has water content, which can dilute the medicinal constituents.

Avoid Shattered Glass

When making infusions, or any time you're pouring hot water into glass, pour slowly! Shocking the glass with abruptly changing temperatures (even glass formulated for use with hot liquids) can lead it to crack or shatter. Avoid using jars or other glass containers that have chips in them, as this can also cause them to shatter when exposed to heat.

Infusion Recipe

This simple infusion recipe works with the majority of plants in this book, but keep in mind it's best used for more delicate plant material, such as flowers and leaves.

YOU'LL NEED:
- 8 ounces water
- 1-2 tablespoons dried herbs or 2-4 tablespoons fresh herbs
- Honey (optional)

1. Bring the water to a boil. While the water is heating, put the herbs in a tea strainer and place them in a mug. Once boiling, pour the water over the herbs. Immediately cover the mug with a plate or lid and allow to steep.

2. After steeping for 10–15 minutes, remove the tea strainer from the water. Drink as is or with honey. Store for up to 1 week in the fridge.

DOSAGE AND STORAGE. Drink one to three servings (1 cup or 8 ounces per serving) per day. The ideal dosage will vary depending on the strength of the plant used and your particular body. Start small and increase as needed.

TRY IT WITH:

Mullein. The leaves dry easily, but you can also use fresh plant material to make an infusion. A hot mullein infusion is great for respiratory health, helping soothe a cold and tame a dry, irritating cough.

Raspberry leaves. You can make an infusion using fresh leaves, if in season, or from dried leaves. This infusion is nutritive and is particularly helpful for those

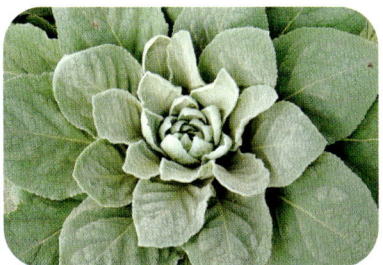

Fresh or dried mullein is excellent in a hot infusion.

in need of uterine support, whether pregnant or looking to ease painful menstrual symptoms.

Yarrow. Yarrow flowers dry well and make an excellent infusion. They can aid in digestion; try a cup of tea before or after a meal to prevent an upset stomach.

Overnight Infusion Recipe

An overnight infusion combines the effects of heat and time to fully extract the medicinal compounds from plant material, creating a very concentrated infusion.

YOU'LL NEED:

- 32 ounces water
- 8 tablespoons dried plant material or 2 large handfuls fresh plant material

1. Bring the water to a boil and place the plant material directly in a heat-safe quart-size jar. Slowly pour the boiling water over the plant material, covering it completely. Cover the jar lightly with a lid.

2. Let the infusion sit overnight at room temperature. The next day, strain out the plant material and enjoy the infusion.

DOSAGE AND STORAGE. Overnight infusions can be drunk like general infusions, 1–3 cups a day as desired. Store in the fridge for up to 1 week.

TRY IT WITH:

Stinging nettle. An overnight infusion is one of the best ways to extract nettle's powerful benefits. A regular infusion will give you a yellow tea, but this overnight infusion will look dark green, even black by morning! This is because of the multitude of compounds and the chlorophyll extracted in this process, resulting in a nutrient-dense preparation that will nourish anyone lucky enough to drink it.

Red clover. This plant is rich in B vitamins along with trace minerals; an overnight infusion of the blossoms can extract even more of those nutritive qualities. Try it with either fresh or dried blossoms.

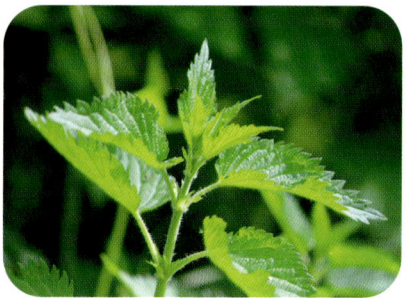

Stinging nettle is rich in calcium, vitamins, iron, and trace minerals, which can be better extracted via an overnight infusion.

Cold Infusion Recipe

Cold infusions are one of the easiest ways to make medicine, no heat or stovetop required—simply steep herbs in cold or room-temperature water, drawing out the plant's medicine gradually. This process is ideal for extracting polysaccharides, the heat-sensitive compounds that form the beneficial mucilage in mucilaginous plants.

YOU'LL NEED:

- 1 cup fresh plant material or ½ cup dried plant material (leaves or flowers are best, but for many plants all parts can be used)

1. Add the plant material to a quart-size jar, crushing it gently to increase the surface area. Add water to fill the jar and completely cover the plant material. Attach the jar lid and allow the infusion to sit at room temperature or in the fridge. (I like it refrigerated for a more refreshing experience when drinking.) It will be ready in about 8 hours.

2. Strain out the plant material before drinking if you wish. And that's it!

DOSAGE AND STORAGE. Cold infusions are cooling and hydrating and can be drunk throughout the day to nourish the body. Drinking 3–4 cups daily is perfect. The strained infusion can be stored in the fridge for up to 1 week.

TRY IT WITH:

Mallow. Mallow is a mucilaginous, soothing plant that is ideal for a cold infusion. This preparation helps ease digestive upset, calm irritation in the gut, and soothe a sore throat and cough. It's especially helpful for cooling the body during the summer months.

Linden. A cold infusion of linden flowers is excellent for mild respiratory ailments and an unsettled stomach. A linden infusion can also be used to help lower a fever and calm the body during or after illness.

Decoctions

A decoction is an herbal preparation made by bringing water and plant material to a rolling boil and maintaining this temperature and intensity to extract compounds from the plant material. This approach is best for fibrous and dense materials, such as mushrooms, barks, and roots. The extended exposure to heat helps break down cell walls and physically break apart tough materials.

For a decoction, I recommend adding the plant material at the beginning, before the water comes to a boil. As a general guideline, keep roots and barks at a rolling boil while covered for about one hour. Some dense, large pieces of plant material might need a few hours, but for most well-chopped materials an hour is perfect.

Herbalism is a sensory experience. If the water is still clear after 45 minutes, this could mean the plant material is not viable, but most times you'll see a distinct color and smell its aroma at this point, letting you know the medicine has been extracted. You can also taste it (once cooled) to be sure. Decoctions can usually be stored out of the fridge for a few days and refrigerated for up to 2 weeks.

Decoction is ideal for tough, fibrous plant material like roots and mushrooms. The extended exposure to heat helps draw out the medicinal and nutritive properties.

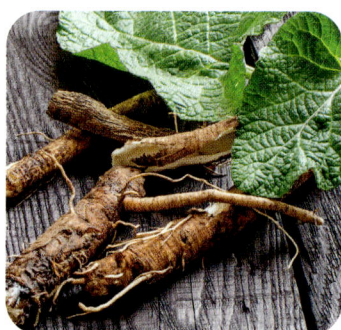
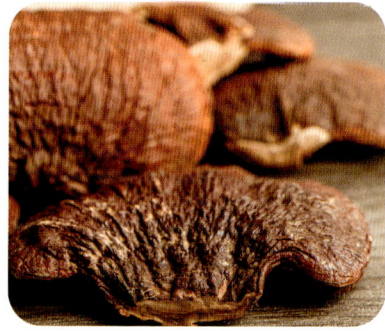

Decoction Recipe

Feel free to adjust the amounts if you'd like a smaller batch: You're aiming for two tablespoons of dried plant material (double that for fresh plants) for every eight ounces of water.

YOU'LL NEED:
- 64 ounces water
- 2 cups dried plant material or 4 well-packed cups fresh plant material

1. Combine the water and plant material in a large pot and place over medium-high heat. Once the mixture begins to steam, cover the pot. When the decoction reaches a rolling boil, set a timer for about 45 minutes. Keep the water at a boil; you may need to adjust the temperature to avoid the pot boiling over. By the end of the time, you'll have a more concentrated medicine.

2. After 45 minutes to an hour, turn off the heat and allow the decoction to cool while covered. Strain out the plant material and store in a lidded jar.

DOSAGE AND STORAGE. Decoctions can be drunk as needed, usually 2–3 cups a day to receive the effects. You can refrigerate your decoction, drink it while still warm, or enjoy it at room temperature. Store in the fridge for up to 2 weeks.

TRY IT WITH:

Reishi. This mushroom benefits from a long boil to break down the cell walls. Try drinking a cup three times a day to nourish the cardiovascular and immune systems. It's also a great bitter for digestion.

Burdock. Try this with fresh burdock roots. The water should turn a light yellow. Drink a cup three times a day to enjoy its diuretic and alterative properties.

Kudzu. A decoction made from the dried roots is mildly sweet and nutritive. It's a helpful tonic to regulate blood pressure and blood sugar, to assist the respiratory system, or to address the symptoms of a hangover.

Tinctures

A tincture is simply an extract of herbs in alcohol, and it is a staple preparation in herbal medicine. Tinctures are shelf stable for about three to five years, but I predict you'll use them well before that. Alcohol is excellent at extracting almost all the healing compounds from plants, helped by the fact that it includes a small amount of water content as well. Pure alcohol is not used for tinctures, as it shouldn't be ingested.

FOLK METHOD

There are two ways to make a tincture, the "technical" way and the "folk" method. Being somewhat of a folk myself, I most often opt for the latter, which involves chopping up and stuffing herbs into a jar and filling the jar completely with alcohol without measuring precise ratios. Because the herbs are so tightly packed, it's best to slowly pour small amounts of alcohol into the jar to avoid air bubbles forming in the plant material.

This more relaxed way of making tinctures creates medicines that are just as effective and useful as those made with specific ratios. As you become more experienced, you'll develop a keen intuition about how to best work with a particular plant.

When making folk tinctures, I typically use high-proof alcohols (between 50 and 85 percent ABV) for barks, roots, and seeds,

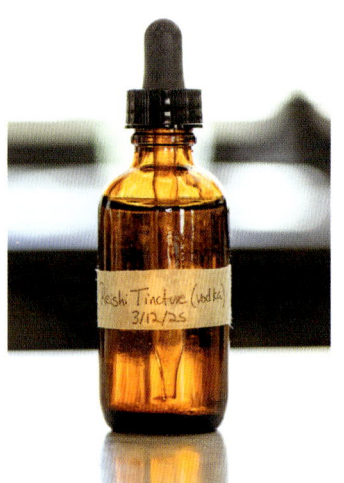

Tinctures are one of the most potent forms of plant medicine.

while lower proof (between 20 and 45 percent ABV) is better for aromatics, leaves, and flowers.

TECHNICAL METHOD: TINCTURE RATIOS

Tinctures can also be made using a more technical approach. On many tinctures, you'll see labels like "1:4 75%" or "1:2 95%." These numbers indicate the ratio of extraction. The first number refers to the weight of the herbs, and the second number refers to the volume of the menstruum—in this case alcohol. If you added 10 ounces of plant material to 40 ounces of alcohol, you would have a 1:4 ratio. The percentage refers to the amount of liquid in the tincture that is alcohol. 75 percent indicates that the liquid in the tincture is 75 percent alcohol and 25 percent water, while 95 percent indicates that the tincture only has 5 percent water. There are many ways to approach tincture ratios, but I generally prefer 95 percent for fresh plants, as they already have some water in them, and 75 percent for dried plants, which need a bit of additional water to rehydrate them.

Weight versus Volume

The first measurement in a tincture ratio, indicating the amount of herb used, is a weight, and the second measurement, indicating the amount of liquid used, is a volume. If we measured our herbs by volume we'd run into an issue: One cup of delicate, lightweight blossoms is a very different amount of plant material than one cup of dense seeds. Measuring by weight solves that problem.

That's a lot of percentages, but let's do one equation using a little shortcut. This shortcut depends on the volume of your jar and assumes that you're using grain alcohol that is 95 percent ABV. For this example, I'll use a 1:2 95% tincture in a 32-ounce jar.

First, take the ratio of 1:2 and add those numbers (1 + 2 = 3), then divide the volume of the jar by this sum: In this case, 32 divided by 3 is 10.66. This is the amount of fresh plant material (in ounces by weight) that can fit inside that jar (yes, it's a lot, but it will fit if chopped and stuffed well).

Now let's determine how much liquid to add. To do that, simply multiply 10.66 by 2, the second half of the ratio. That gives 21.32. A volume of 21.32 ounces of alcohol, which we'll round down to 21 ounces for simplicity, will be needed to finish this tincture.

And that's it for math! This magical little shortcut always works. Technical recipes and ratios like these can be helpful, and there are plenty of online resources if you want to dive deeper into the technical side of tincture making. Now that my ears are smoking, let's make some tinctures.

Tincture Calculator

To calculate the amount of plant material and alcohol needed for a tincture, simply fill in the blanks below. These equations assume you're starting with a grain alcohol that is 95 percent ABV.

FOR FRESH PLANTS

You choose the: **Let's do the math:**

_____   _____ + _____ = _____
Desired weight to volume ratio   First number of ratio   second number of ratio

_____   _____ ÷ _____ = _____
Volume of the jar   Volume of jar in ounces   sum from the line above   amount of plant material in ounces by weight

_____ × _____ = _____
Second number of ratio   amount of plant material   volume of alcohol

FOR DRIED PLANTS

Because dried plants need to be rehydrated, we have the extra step of calculating how much water to add, in addition to the alcohol. To make the math simpler, we'll be cheating a bit and treating the 95 percent ABV grain alcohol as if it's 100 percent. The difference will be negligible in the finished tincture.

You choose the: **Let's do the math:**

_____   _____ + _____ = _____
Desired weight to volume ratio   First number of ratio   second number of ratio

_____   _____ ÷ _____ = _____
Volume of the jar   Volume of jar in ounces   sum from the line above   amount of plant material in ounces by weight

_____ × _____ = _____
Second number of ratio   amount of plant material   volume of liquid

_____ × 0.25 = _____
Total volume of liquid   volume of water needed to rehydrate your plant material

_____ − _____ = _____
Total volume of liquid   volume of water   volume of alcohol

Tincture Recipe

Almost every plant in this book benefits from being made into a tincture. Herbal learning is experiential, so don't be afraid to experiment with different types of alcohol and ratios of plants; you'll develop a better understanding of the plants through the process. (Remember, the proof is double the alcohol by volume; for example a 50 percent ABV alcohol is 100 proof; see page 201).

YOU'LL NEED:

Plant material (fresh or dried)

Alcohol of your choice

1. If you're using dried plant material, rehydrate it by mixing it with a small amount of water (1–2 tablespoons for a 16-ounce tincture, or use the tincture calculator on page 217).

2. Making a tincture couldn't be simpler! Add the plant material to a jar, cover with alcohol, seal the jar, and allow it to steep for about a month at room temperature.

3. After 1 month, strain out and discard the plant material, making sure to label your finished tincture.

DOSAGE AND STORAGE. Most plant tinctures can be taken at a dosage of 2 dropperfuls (20–40 drops; or about 1–2 mL) three times a day, but stronger, more potent plants can be taken at half that dosage (1 dropperful or about ½–1 mL, one or two times a day). Every plant is different and so is every body. Begin at a low dosage and increase as needed as you get a sense of its impact on your system.

When using alcohol, your tincture's shelf life will extend for many years, but I recommend using it within 1–2 years.

TRY IT WITH:

Japanese knotweed. Japanese knotweed root is a powerful medicine that can be used for infections, viral problems throughout the body, and respiratory ailments. A concentrated tincture is the best way to administer this medicine. The finished product is a beautiful blood red color. You can use dried or fresh Japanese knotweed root. If you're using fresh, make sure you chop it the same day as harvesting, as the roots get hard very quickly.

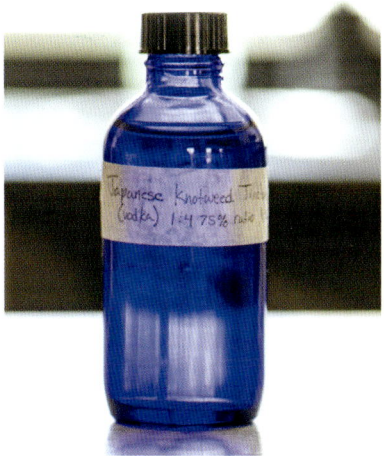

Motherwort. Motherwort is an excellent nervine that relaxes and nourishes the nervous system. In tincture form, you can take this medicine at any time to ease stress. Try making this tincture using the folk method: Simply stuff your jar with motherwort and top with a low-proof alcohol. Motherwort is a beautiful green color when fully extracted.

Tips for Making Tinctures

- If you're using dried plant material, you'll need to add some water to rehydrate it. If you're using the folk method, about 2 tablespoons of water for a 16-ounce tincture is a good guideline. If you're using the ratio approach, refer to the calculator on page 217 to determine the amount of water needed.

- Dried herbs can sometimes absorb liquid over the first 24 hours. When using dried herbs, check your tinctures the first day or two to see if you need to add more liquid to ensure all the plant material remains submerged.

- Make sure your tinctures are always free of air bubbles and that the ingredients are well broken down to facilitate the extraction process.

- The more plant material you include, the more concentrated the tincture will be.

- When making folk tinctures, high-proof alcohol is better for tough and fibrous material such as bark and roots, whereas lower-proof alcohol is best for leaves, shoots, and flowers.

- Finished tinctures can be decanted into amber dropper bottles, which makes them easy to dose and protects them from light.

- Tinctures are best stored away from direct light and high heat—a closed cabinet is ideal.

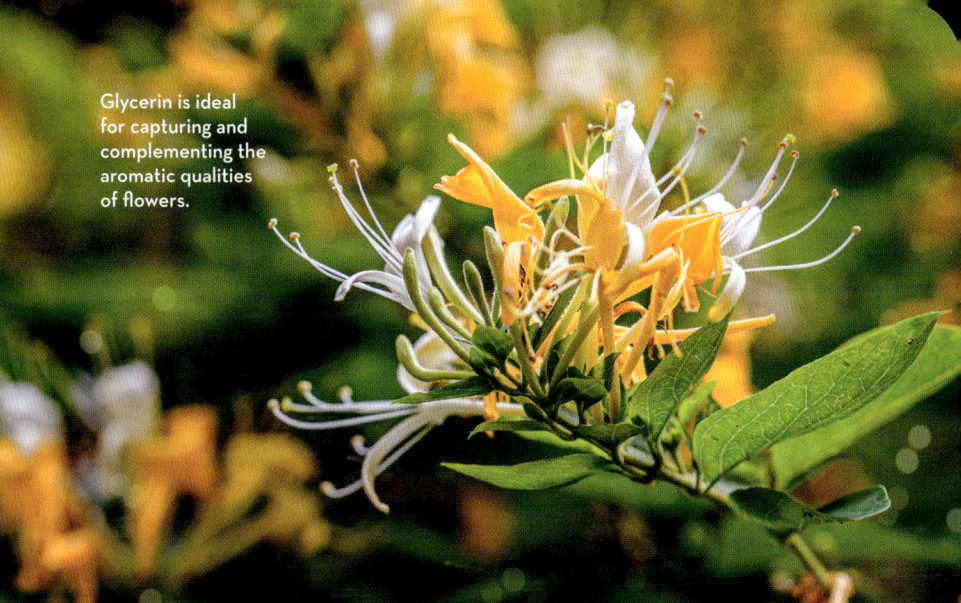

Glycerin is ideal for capturing and complementing the aromatic qualities of flowers.

Glycerin Extracts

An herbal glycerin is made by extracting plant material with vegetable glycerin, a liquid made from plant oils such as palm, coconut, and soy. Vegetable glycerin is sweet, viscous, and efficient at pulling medicine out of certain crushed roots and many leaves and flowers. While vegetable glycerin extracts many compounds, alcohol tinctures are often more efficient. It's best to reserve glycerin for thin and delicate plant material.

    Glycerin is great for those who can't consume alcohol but want the convenience of a tincture in a dropper bottle. Its sweet flavor also makes it a favorite for children. Glycerin can help them swallow plants that are less agreeable, which, depending on the child, could mean all plants.

Glycerin Extract Recipe

This recipe has two different options for preparation, depending on how much time you have. The first is a heatless method that allows the plant material to infuse for a month. The second uses boiling water over low heat to extract the medicinal compounds over the course of a few hours.

Sometimes I like to combine methods and allow the mixture to infuse for an additional two to three weeks after heating and before I've strained it.

YOU'LL NEED:

- Enough dry or fresh plant material to completely fill a container (adjust the jar size depending on how much material)
- 16 ounces vegetable glycerin; be sure to purchase food-grade glycerin

1. Add the herbs to a jar (be sure to use a heat-safe jar if using the boiling-water method). If using dried herbs, add 1–2 tablespoons of water to slightly rehydrate the plant material. This is just enough to rehydrate but not water down the tincture.

2. Pour in the glycerin, using a fork or spoon to stir up the material, ensuring no air bubbles form. Continue stirring and pouring to the top of the jar, making sure all plant material is completely covered.

Option One: Heatless Method

3. Cover the jar and allow it to sit for 30 days at room temperature, straining out the plant material at the end of that time.

Option Two: Boiling-Water Method

4. Place the sealed jar in a pot and add water to the pot until the the water comes halfway up the jar. If you prefer, place a steamer basket or metal rack in the pot before adding the jar, to prevent it from being in direct contact with the bottom of the pot.

5. Place the pot on the stove over very low heat, keeping the water at a simmer for 6–8 hours. If the pot is tall enough, cover it with a lid to increase the heat. Keep an eye on the pot, ensuring that the water doesn't begin to boil and that the water level hasn't decreased. Add more water as needed.

6. After the time has elapsed, allow the mixture to cool. Once cool, strain out the plant material and store.

DOSAGE AND STORAGE. Glycerin extracts have a shelf life of about 1 year. They can be taken in the same dosages as alcohol tinctures: 2 dropperfuls (20–40 drops; 1–2 mL) three times a day, or a half dosage (1 dropperful; ½–1 mL) one or two times a day for particularly potent plants.

TRY IT WITH:

Linden. Linden flower works well in a glycerin extract as it is not overly fibrous, releases its aromatic medicine easily, and doesn't take long to extract.

Mimosa. Glycerin is a great base menstruum to capture the aromatic qualities of mimosa. The resulting medicine is a calming nervine to help ease anxiety and daily stress.

Honeysuckle. Glycerin is the ideal menstruum to capture the delicate, aromatic qualities of honeysuckle. The resulting medicine can help with respiratory issues.

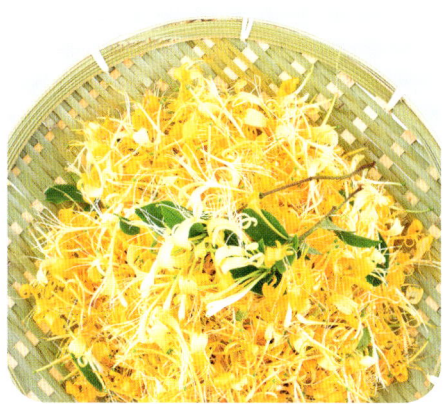

Glycerin extractions add a sweet note to your medicine making, which is a perfect pairing with honeysuckle.

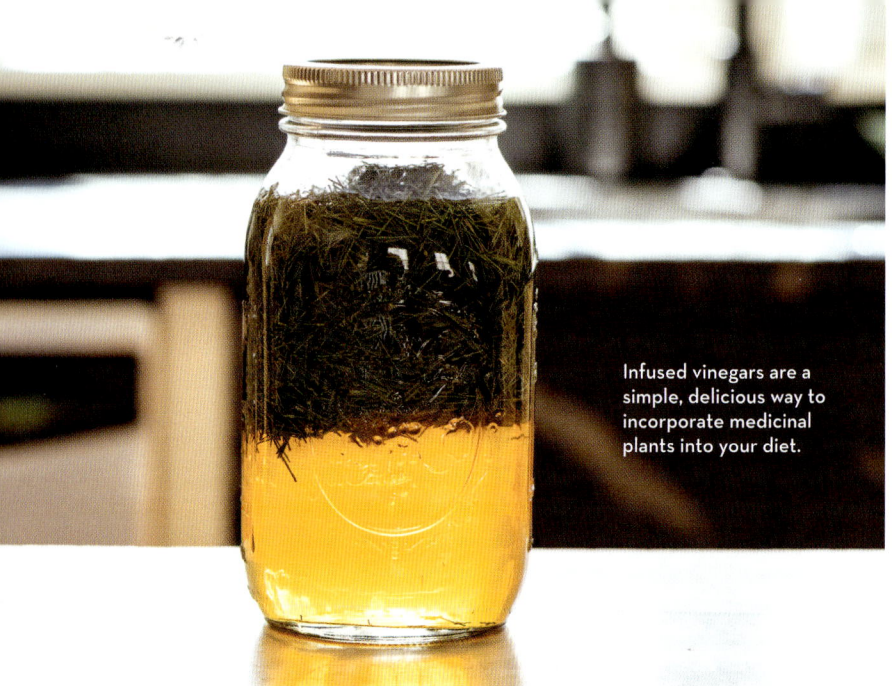

Infused vinegars are a simple, delicious way to incorporate medicinal plants into your diet.

Herbal Vinegars

Apple cider vinegar infusions are delicious and potent ways to make medicine; they're a great example of food as medicine. Apple cider vinegar helps extract flavors and aromatic compounds as well as vitamins and minerals from nutritive herbs. It has an affinity for the digestive system and respiratory system, acting as an expectorant to help clear congestion. The perfect bridge between medicine and food, many vinegar-based preparations have a permanent home in my medicine cabinet.

Though there are many kinds of vinegar, apple cider vinegar is preferred for medicinal use (see page 199) as it offers health benefits of its own and is readily available.

Herbal Vinegar Recipe

Herbal vinegars are a delicious fusion of food and medicine. And the best part is that they are incredibly simple to make.

YOU'LL NEED:

- 1 large handful of plant material, dried or fresh
- 32 ounces apple cider vinegar
- 1 cup honey (optional)

1. Using scissors or a knife, cut the plant material into small pieces, about $1/4$ inch in size. Add the plant material to a quart-size jar and pour in the vinegar, making sure all the plant material is covered. Put the lid on and allow the mixture to steep for a month before straining and using.

2. For more respiratory support, add the honey to the finished vinegar. This makes an *oxymel*, a honey-and-vinegar combination that is great for any respiratory ailment.

DOSAGE AND STORAGE. Vinegars can be taken in any amount you prefer and can be used for pickling and making salad dressings, and even drunk as straight shots.

TRY IT WITH:

Pine. Pine vinegar is great for getting a dose of antioxidants, aromatics, and vitamin C in winter. I like to add it to sauces and dressings and even make herbal shrubs with it because of its tasty pine aroma. Pine vinegar helps stimulate digestion in winter and encourage circulation, helping clean out any congestion.

Garlic mustard. Use roots, stems, and leaves for this recipe; just make sure to mince the garlic mustard material. You'll need about 3 cups of plant material for 32 ounces of vinegar. Want a little more kick? Throw in two hot peppers and you'll be blowing your nose for a week.

Honeysuckle. The blooms can be infused in vinegar to bring out their soothing and antibacterial properties. This sweet and tart vinegar is great for cough and congestion as well as soothing a sore throat.

Herbal Steams

An herbal steam is made by bringing water to a boil and adding aromatic herbs. The resulting vapor is rich in essential oils, aromatic compounds that are naturally antibacterial and antifungal and can relax the nervous system, among other actions. Herbal steams are inhaled for a total of 10 to 15 minutes. When paired with deep breathing, they can help ease congestion, releasing phlegm and clearing the sinuses.

In addition to being a powerful decongestant, an herbal steam can be an excellent way to relax and de-stress. Take the opportunity to practice mindful breathing, inhaling and exhaling slowly and deeply, to fully benefit from the medicinal compounds and promote both physical and mental wellness.

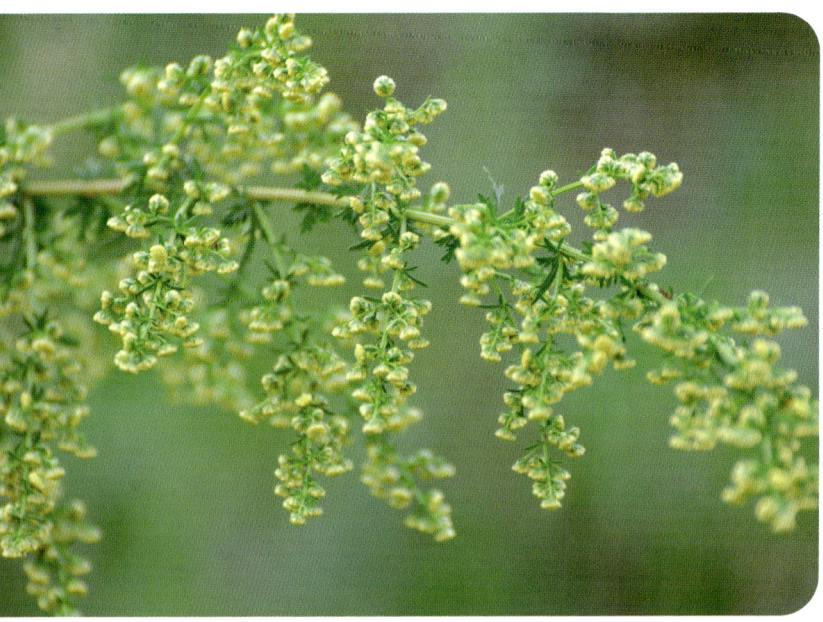

Herbal Steam Recipe

A word of caution: Steam is, obviously, incredibly hot, so be careful as you breathe. You want to inhale the warm, aromatic steam as it rises and cools, not stick your whole face directly into the pot and end up with a scalded nose. Expect to cough a bit if you're congested. This is a good thing and will help you breathe easily again!

YOU'LL NEED:
- 1 cup dried herbs or a handful of fresh stems and leaves
- Towel

1. Bring a pot of water to a boil over medium heat. When the water is boiling, remove the pot from the stove and place it on a trivet or heat-safe surface somewhere you can comfortably breathe the steam.

2. Add the herbs, mixing them into the water. Then cover your head and the pot with a towel, inhaling deeply through the nose and mouth for a few minutes before uncovering your head to take a break. Repeat the process as needed until the steam stops rising.

TRY IT WITH:

Sweet Annie. The oils in this plant are antibacterial and antimicrobial, helping with infections in the respiratory system and sinuses.

Bee balm. The pungent oils and thyme-like aroma of this plant are perfect for an herbal steam. I like to use this for clearing sinus congestion in wintertime.

Pine. Easy to forage year-round, pine needles make a great herbal steam. They can take the edge off of a headache and ease tension, as well as clear congestion in the chest.

Topical Medicines

The medicinal value of plants isn't limited to internal use. The following preparations are all applied externally. Some are designed to treat skin issues, such as bug bites, cuts and scrapes, or rashes, while others offer deeper healing by supporting lymphatic drainage or even aiding in sleep. External medicines can be one of the most approachable ways to begin using plants and herbs.

POULTICES

A poultice is made when a plant is applied directly to the skin. Usually the plant is fresh, but occasionally it can be dried. Most of the plants used for this purpose are vulneraries, helping stimulate wound healing, and many are anti-inflammatory to help relieve bug bites, rash, heat irritation, and the like. Some plants used in poultices are also drawing, pulling out stingers, splinters, and venom from ant and bug bites. Poultices can also be used for deeper ailments, such as sprains and pain from bruising and sore muscles, and are applied in the same manner.

HERBAL OILS

Herbal oils are a great way to capture the aromatic and skin-soothing qualities of a plant. Oil is a fat typically derived from seeds. It pulls the essential oils, also known as volatile oils, out of plants, creating a wonderfully aromatic medicine that can be rubbed on the body for therapeutic use. These volatile oils are actually a defense mechanism in plants and are inherently antibacterial, antimicrobial, and antifungal. They also have an affinity for our respiratory and digestive systems. Any type of aromatic plant, especially ones that are used in the culinary world, such as thyme or rosemary, works well as an oil.

Essential Oils

Commercially available essential oils are made using steam distillation to extract the plant's volatile oils, making them incredibly concentrated. The infusion method in this book won't be as potent, but you'll still benefit from the plant's medicinal properties (without needing to purchase any complicated distillation equipment!).

Humans have a fascinating part of the brain called the limbic system, which is activated by smell and is responsible for memory recall, feelings of nostalgia, and emotion. If you've ever caught a familiar scent—your mother's perfume, the scent of your first car—and been instantly transported to an old memory, you've experienced the limbic system at work. Aromatherapy works by using scent to regulate the nervous system. By associating smells with calmness, peace, and safety, we can access those feelings even in times of stress. When you infuse your own oils with aromatic botanicals, you can harness not only their medicinal effects but also the brain's powerful recall of smell.

HERBAL HAIR WASH

Hair washes don't just nourish your hair! These plant-infused washes allow our skin, nails, hair, and scalp to experience the beneficial qualities of whichever medicinal herb is used. The act of washing your hair with an herbal hair wash is soothing and healing in and of itself.

Poultice Recipe

This is one of the easiest ways to administer an herbal medicine, especially if you're out in the forest or field!

YOU'LL NEED:

- 1 handful of clean fresh or dried plant material
- Gauze or Band-Aid (optional)

1. Crush the plant material with a mortar and pestle until it forms a paste. If using dried plant material, add a small amount of water until a paste forms. If out in the field, simply chew the fresh plant material to break it down.

2. Apply the paste to the afflicted area. Hold it in place for several minutes or wrap it with gauze or a Band-Aid to secure it. Once it dries or you feel relief, you can remove it. This process can be repeated as many times as necessary.

TRY IT WITH:

Chickweed. The leaves of this plant are high in water content, so it's easily transformed into a cooling poultice that can work well on bug bites, rashes, and even eczema.

Plantain. A plantain poultice is one of my favorites for bee stings, splinters, bug bites, and rashes. Once when I was stung by a bee, I immediately crushed some nearby plantain leaf and applied it to my ankle. Within about 10 seconds the pain was gone. You can do this with dried plantain leaf as well: Simply rehydrate it with a splash of water before applying.

Yarrow. This plant is a powerful styptic, meaning that it stops bleeding. Historically, soldiers used it on the battlefield, applying it to their wounds. Use the (clean!) flowers to create a poultice for scrapes and cuts—you'll be amazed at how effectively it works.

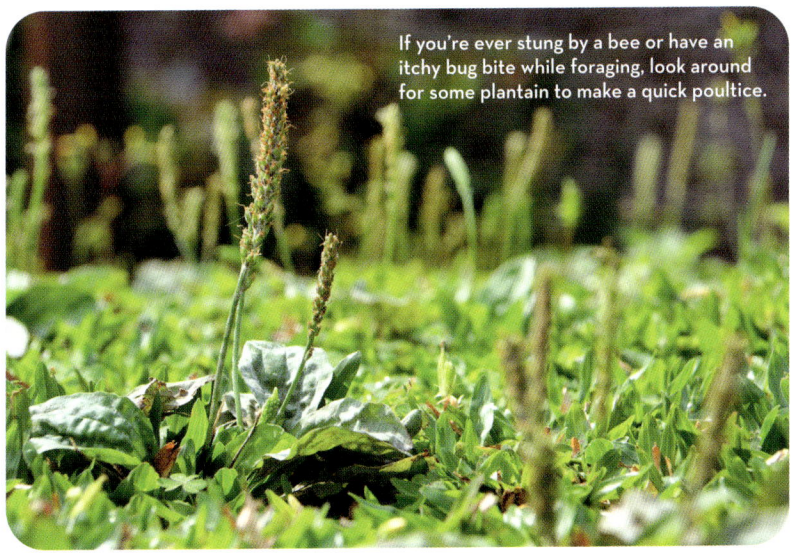

If you're ever stung by a bee or have an itchy bug bite while foraging, look around for some plantain to make a quick poultice.

Herbal Oil Recipe

Herbal oils are best made with dried herbs. This recipe includes two options: a heatless version that allows plant materials to infuse over the course of a month, and a speedier boiling-water method.

The water content of fresh plant material can leave oil prone to spoilage, so if you must use fresh plants, make sure to crush them well, use the boiling-water method, and store the oil in the refrigerator.

YOU'LL NEED:

- 2 cups dried plant material
- 16 ounces extra-virgin olive oil

1. Crush the dried plant material well and add it to a jar (be sure to select a heat-safe jar if using the boiling-water method). Pour the oil over the plant material, stirring to avoid clumping and air bubbles. Fill the jar to the top, covering all of the plant material.

Option One: Heatless Method

2. Attach the lid to the jar and store it in a cool, dark place at room temperature for 1 month to allow the oil to infuse. After a month, strain out the plant material and the oil will be ready for use.

Option Two: Boiling-Water Method

3. Heat accelerates the infusion process. Place the sealed jar in a pot and add water to the pot until the water comes halfway up the jar. If you prefer, place a steamer basket or metal rack in the pot before adding the jar, to prevent it from being in direct contact with the bottom of the pot.

4. Place the pot over very low heat and keep the water at a simmer for 6–8 hours. If the pot is large enough, cover it with a lid to increase the heat. Keep an eye on it, making sure it doesn't boil and that the water level hasn't decreased. Add more water as needed.

5. You'll know the oil is ready when the aroma has changed or the oil has taken on the color of the plant material. When the infusion process is complete, remove the jar and allow it to cool slowly before straining out the plant material. Decant the oil into smaller jars if desired. Be sure to label them appropriately.

USAGE AND STORAGE. Rub a small amount into your skin as needed or use in cooking, depending on the plant. Herbal oils made with dried herbs can be shelf stable for up to 1 year.

TRY IT WITH:

Violet. Made with dried violet leaves and flowers, this massage oil can help stimulate lymphatic flow and drainage. Lymph is found throughout the body, especially around the armpits, neck, and breasts, and makes up a key part of our immune system. When you drain your lymph nodes and stimulate flow, you help your body clean out pathogens and support your immune system.

Mugwort. An oil-based infusion utilizes mugwort leaves' aromatic and warming scent. Associated with the moon and sleep, mugwort can help regulate sleep cycles and relax the nervous system. This oil can be applied around the temples or on the wrists before bed. It's also a great massage oil!

Plantain. This oil is a great remedy for bug bites and rashes and stimulates healing of cuts and scrapes. Due to its pulling effect, it can also help pull out splinters and bee stingers.

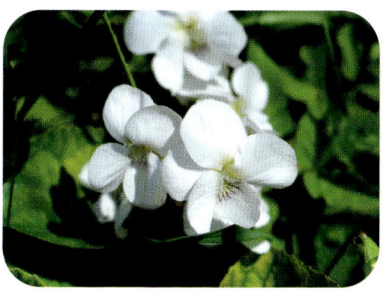

continued on next page

Herbal Oil Recipe, continued

Mullein. The flowers can be infused into oil and used in the ears to soothe earaches and inflammation. The flower-infused oil can also be used topically to soothe irritated and itchy skin.

Red clover. Herbal oil infused with dried blossoms is excellent for lymphatic massage and stimulating lymphatic drainage.

Yarrow. Infusing yarrow flowers into oil captures their vulnerary properties. I love using this oil to accelerate the healing process for cuts, scrapes, and burns; it's also excellent for keeping skin hydrated.

Pine. Pine needles and bark can be made into an invigorating and refreshing oil infusion that stimulates circulation in cold temperatures. Applied to the temples, it can help clear congestion and ease tension headaches.

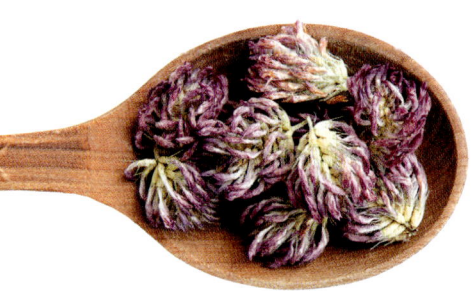

It's best to use dried plants for oil infusions, as too much moisture can lead to mold or spoilage.

Herbal Hair Wash Recipe

This recipe is made in the same way you would make a tea, but instead of ingesting it you apply it to the scalp to nourish the skin and hair.

To use, pour the rinse slowly onto your scalp, massaging as you do so. You want the liquid to be absorbed by your skin and hair follicles, so don't wash it off with water. Let air-dry and repeat as desired.

YOU'LL NEED:

- 32 ounces water
- 6 tablespoons dried plant material

1. Add the water to a pot and bring to a boil over medium-high heat. Once the water is boiling, add the plant material, stirring before covering. Gently boil for about 10 minutes.

2. Turn off the heat and leave the pot on the stovetop to steep and cool down.

3. Once the liquid has cooled enough to touch, strain out the plant material and pour the hair wash into a jar.

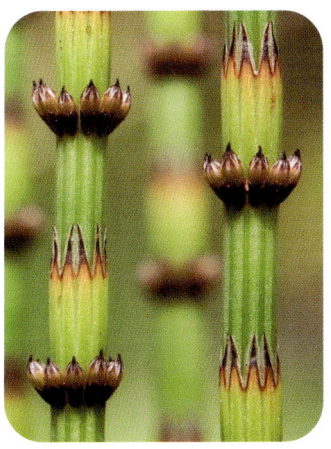

STORAGE. This will be good in the fridge for about 2 weeks, but I often use 32 ounces in one go.

TRY IT WITH:

Horsetail. Horsetail makes an excellent wash that encourages hair growth. Use once or twice per week for best results.

Stinging nettle. The silica and trace minerals in nettle promote hair growth and cleanse the scalp, which can help with conditions such as eczema and psoriasis.

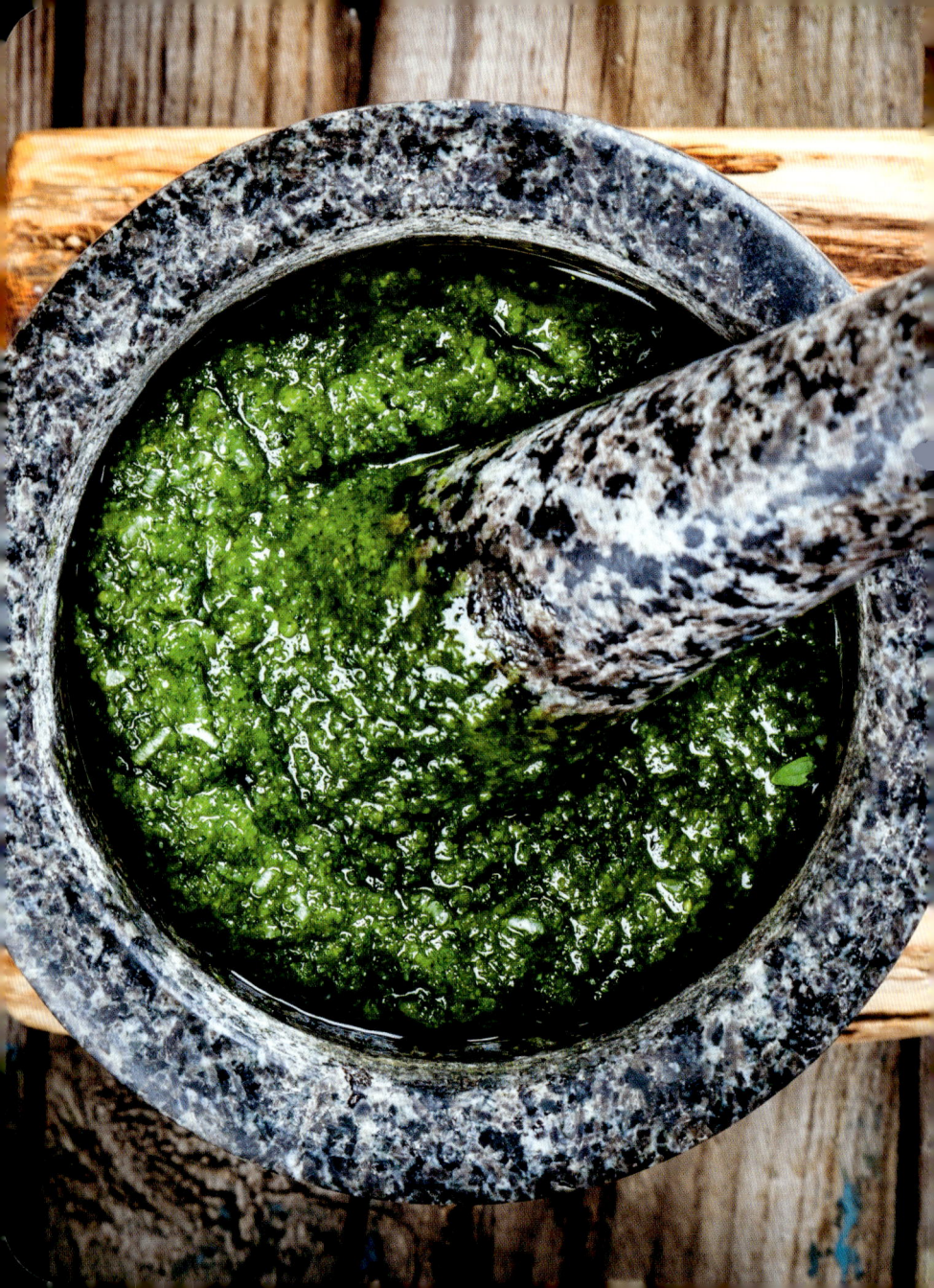

CHAPTER 9

FOOD
as Medicine

We've explored numerous ways to make plant medicine, but we can also enjoy the healing benefits of plants through food. In this chapter you'll find some simple, approachable recipes to help you incorporate medicinal plants into your everyday eating—from pesto to soda!

Medicinal Foods

Our food is medicine. So many of the plants mentioned in this book can be used as food or as complements to food with their flavors and health benefits. The distinction between food and medicine is often arbitrary, and this is particularly true with medicinal plants.

Plants have been used as medicine for thousands of years by people all over the world. In many instances there has been little, if any, differentiation between food and medicine. Most of the plants mentioned in this book are popular as wild foods but, depending on the part used or stage of ripeness when they are harvested, also have medicinal qualities.

While the plants in this book make great acute remedies, incorporating the healing power of plants into your regular diet is a powerful way to benefit from their medicinal qualities more consistently. Whether in syrups, jams, and seasoning powders or simply as dried herbs, the more we consume these plants on a regular basis, the more we will see changes in our health and well-being.

The Power of Honey

Far more than just a tasty sweetener, honey is antibacterial, anti-inflammatory, and antioxidant. It's the perfect collision of food and medicine. Taking a teaspoon internally is great for a sore or scratchy throat (particularly when infused with bee balm or pine), but you can also use it to sweeten your tea, drizzle it on oatmeal or cornbread, incorporate it into baking, or mix it into dressings and marinades.

Wild Rose Honey

Herbal honeys use minimal heat to extract the aromatic qualities, flavors, and medicinal constituents from plants. Wild rose is the perfect example—this honey captures its aromatic qualities and can be used to sweeten teas or add some sweetness anywhere else you'd enjoy it.

YOU'LL NEED:

- 2 cups dried rose petals
- 16 ounces honey

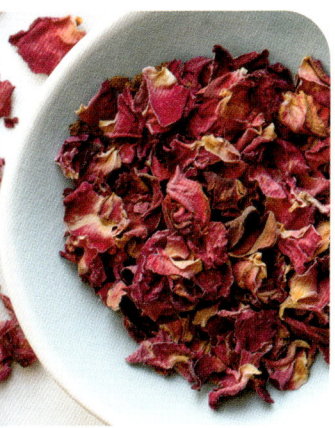

Try adding rose honey to desserts, mixing it into yogurt or oatmeal, or using it to sweeten anything from your morning coffee to a glass of sweet tea.

1. Lightly crush the petals to increase the surface area and release their aroma. You don't want to powder them completely, as they will then be nearly impossible to separate from the honey; simply break them up a bit.

2. Add the petals to a jar and pour the honey slowly over them while mixing with a spatula to avoid air bubbles. If your honey is too solid to pour, you can put the jar in warm water until it has softened sufficiently. Ensure the honey covers the petals completely.

3. Store the honey at room temperature. After 30 days it will be ready to use.

4. The petals can be eaten with the honey, or they can be strained out. The straining process for honey is tedious but doable—just use a strainer with relatively large holes.

STORAGE. This honey will be shelf stable without refrigeration indefinitely, as honey is one of the most shelf-stable foods there is!

continued on next page

Wild Rose Honey, continued

TRY IT WITH:

Bee balm. Bee balm honey is a great remedy for sore throat and cough. If you're using fresh flowers, pack down 2 cups of flowers, then chop them well before combining with honey. The finished honey is great for flavoring teas or as its own medicine (taken by the teaspoon if you have a sweet tooth like me).

Mimosa. Mimosa blooms in honey create a sweet, aromatic medicine that calms the mind and soul. The flowers are fluffy and take up much less volume once they've been crushed, so have some extra. You'll end up with a wonderfully pink honey sure to help you beat the blues. Fresh blooms are ideal, as they are far more aromatic than dried flowers.

Pine. It's best to use pine needles instead of bark or resin, which can be harder to break apart and require a bit of heat to extract their medicinal properties. Chop up your needles well and cover with honey for a refreshing and sweet remedy for cough and cold symptoms. Fresh needles are preferred.

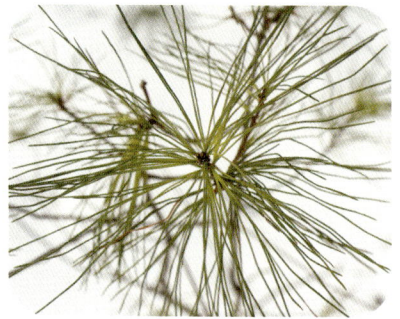

Fresh pine needles infused into honey make a great winter cough remedy.

Linden. Linden flowers' aromatic qualities shine in an herbal honey and make a great addition to an evening tea. This nervine tastes and smells delicious, and can help you ease any tension from the day and drift into sleep in the evening. These can be used fresh or dried.

Garlic mustard. This is pungent and powerful, with the soothing effects of honey complementing garlic mustard's flavor and aroma. Together, they help loosen congestion and warm the body. This is a great medicine to prep in summer while the plant is plentiful, storing it up for use in winter. Fresh plant parts are ideal for preserving the pungent scent.

Bee Balm Salt

Bee balm is rich in volatile oils such as thymol, giving it a strong aroma. All species have this feature and can be used in this recipe, but I've found Monarda punctata, *which grows through the southeastern US, to be the strongest.*

Bee balm–infused salt can be used to add a savory, aromatic flavor to your cooking. I prefer to make salt with fresh herbs, but dried can also be used. If you use dried herbs, the finished result will be more of a seasoning blend than an herbal salt.

YOU'LL NEED:

- 4 cups packed fresh bee balm flowers or 3 cups dried flowers
- 2½ cups salt, plus more if needed

1. Place the flowers in a food processor and blend briefly until well chopped.

2. Add the salt. It will absorb any excess moisture from the blooms and extract the flavor and aroma.

3. Blend again briefly; don't turn the salt to powder, just combine everything well. If the mixture seems too wet, add a bit more salt, mixing well.

4. Store the finished salt in a jar at room temperature or in the fridge if you notice too much moisture.

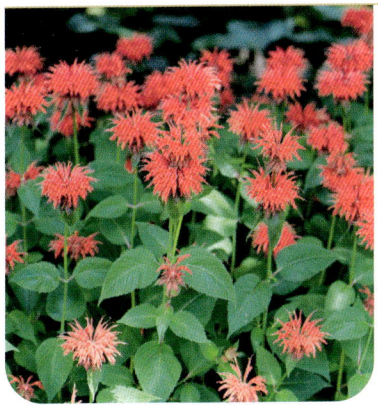

STORAGE. Herbal salts can be stored at room temperature for up to 1 year.

TRY IT WITH:

Garlic mustard. This pungent salt will help clear the sinuses and add a delicious mix of garlic and brassica flavor to any dish. The leaves and flowering heads are best for this purpose, as the roots can be a bit too fibrous to mix with salt.

Chickweed and Wild Greens Pesto

This recipe is a great way to integrate chickweed into your diet and benefit from its medicinal qualities. This recipe is very flexible, so feel free to include whatever wild or cultivated greens you'd prefer. I've added dandelion and purslane, or arugula and spinach. It's really your choice!

YOU'LL NEED:
- 1 handful fresh chickweed
- 2 handfuls greens of choice (or mix two varieties)
- 1 cup fresh basil
- ¾ cup extra-virgin olive oil
- 2 tablespoons lemon juice
- ¾ cup toasted pine nuts
- 2 garlic cloves
- Salt and freshly ground black pepper

1. Place the chickweed, additional greens, basil, oil, and lemon juice in a blender, food processor, or mortar and pestle. Pulse or pound until coarsely chopped and well combined.

2. Add the pine nuts and garlic. Blend again until you've achieved a smooth, well-combined mixture.

3. Once well blended, add salt and pepper to taste.

STORAGE. This is great as a topping and as a dip for crackers and other crunchy foods. Store in the refrigerator for up to 3 weeks.

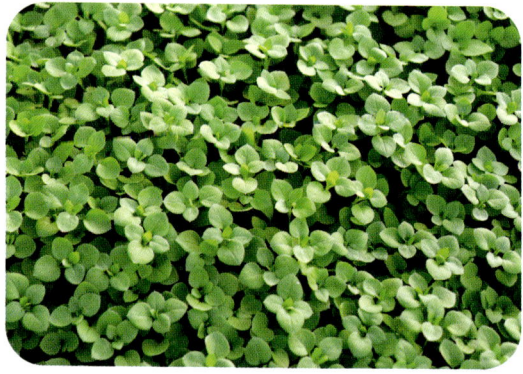

Sumac "Lemonade"

Sumac berries, thanks to their citrusy flavor, have long been used to make a lemonade-like drink. All you need are the berries and water, with a sweetener optional. This recipe is rich in vitamin C and helps cool down the body, especially in the summer heat.

YOU'LL NEED:

- 64 ounces water
- 3 clusters fresh sumac berries, or about 1½ cups dried berries
- 3 tablespoons sugar or honey (optional)
- Salt (optional)

1. Add the water to a pot and bring to a boil over medium-high heat. Add the sumac berries once the water is at a rolling boil.

2. Cover and let simmer for 5 minutes before turning off the heat. Leave the pot on the stovetop to allow the residual heat to continue extracting flavor from the berries.

3. If desired, add the sweetener while the liquid is still warm, then let cool completely, strain out the berries, and store the mixture in a jar or pitcher. I sometimes add a small pinch of salt with each serving to balance the flavor and support hydration.

STORAGE. The lemonade will last for 1–2 weeks refrigerated.

You can use the sumac berries fresh or dried, depending on the season and what you have on hand.

Honeysuckle Soda

My personal obsession with sodas has left me experimenting with all the aromatic plants I encounter, but honeysuckle soda is a favorite.

YOU'LL NEED:

- 2 cups water
- 1½ cups sugar (your choice of sugar; I like panela, a raw brown sugar cone popular in Latin America)
- 4 cups fresh, well-washed honeysuckle flowers; substitute 1½ cups dried flowers if you prefer
- Sparkling water

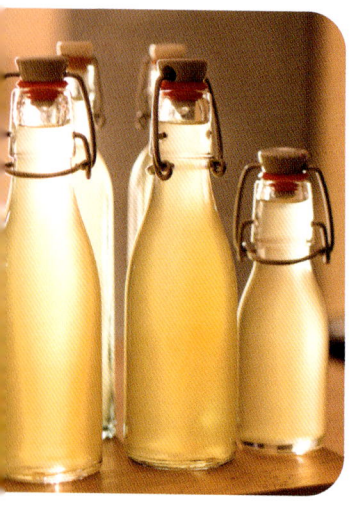

MAKE THE SYRUP

1. Put the water and sugar in a pot, place over medium heat, and simmer until the sugar is well dissolved.

2. Add the flowers and immediately cover the pot. Let the mixture simmer, covered, for about 5 minutes before turning off the heat.

3. Allow the syrup to steep with the lid on until cooled. Once it's fully cool, strain out the honeysuckle.

STORAGE. The finished syrup can be kept in a jar in the fridge for 1 week.

MAKE THE SODA

1. Add some syrup to sparkling water and stir. You can experiment with how much syrup you like, but my preferred ratio is 3 ounces of syrup to 7 ounces of sparkling water. Enjoy!

TRY IT WITH:

Elderflower. Fresh or dried elderflower make a nice, refreshing tonic with immune-supporting benefits.

Rose. Dried petals are best to really get the aromatic properties, and I love the rich pink color of this soda. Garnish with more rose petals!

Linden. Linden flowers are great for a soda and can be used fresh or dried.

Symptom Guide

While herbs aren't cure-alls that can magically heal every ailment without your addressing larger issues of lifestyle and well-being, it's helpful to know which herbs to reach for when you're experiencing illness. In the list below, I've paired common health issues with plants that can offer support. If you're struggling with a particular symptom, you can start here and then read up on the full plant profile to see if it could prove useful.

As always, remember that everybody is different and our systems all react differently to both illness and plant medicine. Listen to your body, consult a healthcare professional when needed, and start with a low dosage when working with a new herb.

Anxiety and sleep problems. Mugwort, motherwort, wild rose, mimosa, linden, reishi

Congestion and cough. Sweet Annie, garlic mustard, Japanese knotweed, mullein, violet, elderberry, bee balm, honeysuckle, pine

Cuts and scrapes. Plantain, yarrow

Digestive upset. Mugwort, violet, mallow

Headache and pain relief. Kudzu, wild lettuce

Immune boost. Spanish needle, elderberry, Oregon grape, reishi

Lymphatic flow. Cleavers, violet

Reproductive wellness. Mugwort, red clover, motherwort, red raspberry

Sore throat. Sweet Annie, elderberry, bee balm, honeysuckle, sumac, reishi

Vitamin and mineral deficiency. Dandelion, chickweed, burdock, red clover, Spanish needle, horsetail, stinging nettle, sumac

RESOURCES

Below are some websites, schools, books, and general resources for learning more about herbal medicine. I personally know many of these educators and programs and can vouch for the amazing work they do providing educational materials that are easy to understand, comprehensive, and valuable for helping us learn about the plants that surround us. There are herbal schools, weekend courses, individual classes, apprenticeships, and so much more out there. Once you get your head in a book, walk through the forest, or meet new friends, you'll be immersed in the abundant resources and community that surround herbal medicine.

BOOKS

Foraging and Feasting: A Field Guide & Wild Food Cookbook by Dina Falconi

Iwígara: American Indian Ethnobotanical Traditions and Science by Enrique Salmón

Peterson Field Guide to Medicinal Plants and Herbs of Eastern and Central North America by Steven Foster and James A. Duke

Southeast Medicinal Plants: Identify, Harvest, and Use 106 Wild Herbs for Health and Wellness by CoreyPine Shane

Wild Plants I Have Known . . . and Eaten by Russ Cohen

Wild Remedies: How to Forage Healing Foods and Craft Your Own Herbal Medicine by Rosalee de la Forêt and Emily Han

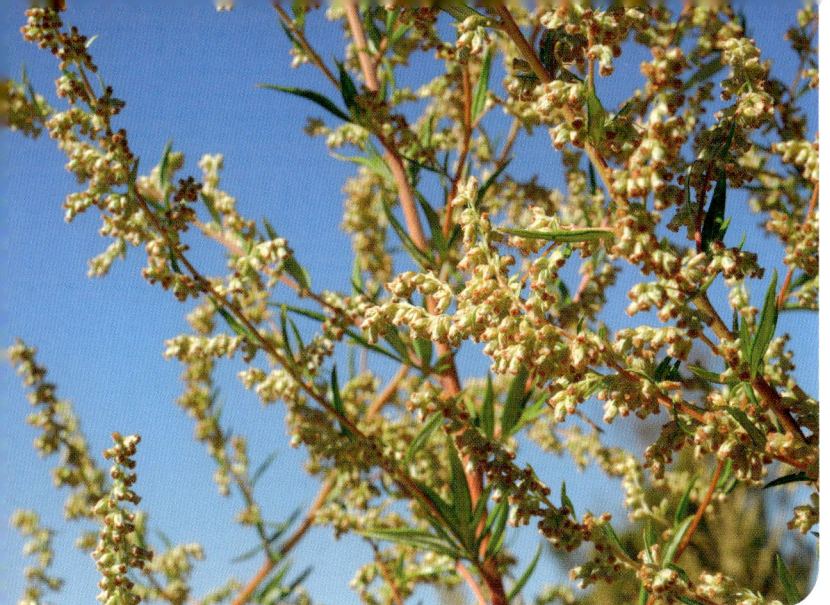

ONLINE EDUCATIONAL PROGRAMS AND RESOURCES

Chestnut School of Herbal Medicine
https://chestnutherbs.com

Herbal Academy
https://theherbalacademy.com

Herbalista
https://herbalista.org

The People's Medicine School
https://rootworkherbals.com/pmsregistration

Wild Ginger Community Herbal Center
https://wildgingerherbalcenter.com

INDEX

A

Achillea millefolium. See yarrow (*Achillea millefolium*)
adaptogens, 188
Albizia julibrissin. See mimosa (*Albizia julibrissin*)
alcohol, 200–201
allergies, 197
Alliaria petiolata. See garlic mustard (*Alliaria petiolata*)
alteratives
  burdock, 103, 104
  Japanese knotweed, 84
  red clover, 107, 108
alternate leaves, 33
analgesics
  pine, 182, 183
  wild lettuce, 111, 112
anatomy of plants, 28–35
anthelmintics, mugwort, 79
antibacterials
  bee balm, 161, 162
  elderberry, 136, 137–138
  garlic mustard, 75, 76
  honeysuckle, 165, 166
  sumac, 173, 175
  sweet Annie, 71
antibiotics
  Oregon grape, 157, 158
  Spanish needle, 115, 116
antifungals, black walnut, 147, 148
anti-inflammatories
  Japanese knotweed, 84, 85
  stinging nettle, 152, 153
  violet, 99, 100

antimalarials, sweet Annie, 71, 72
antimicrobials
  elderberry, 136, 137–138
  Oregon grape, 157, 158
antiparasitics, black walnut, 147, 148
antispasmodics, mugwort, 79, 81
antitussives, honeysuckle, 165, 166
antivirals
  Japanese knotweed, 84, 85
  reishi, 186, 187–188
anxiolytics
  linden, 191, 192
  mimosa, 178
  wild rose, 131, 132
apps, plant ID, 28
Arctium lappa. See burdock (*Arctium lappa*)
Artemisia annua. See sweet Annie (*Artemisia annua*)
Artemisia vulgaris. See mugwort (*Artemisia vulgaris*)
Artemisinin, 72, 73
  See also sweet Annie (*Artemisia annua*)
astringents
  cleavers, 59
  Oregon grape, 157, 158
  raspberry, 169, 170
  sumac, 173, 175
  wild rose, 131, 132–133
Avena sativa. See oat (*Avena sativa*)

B

bags, 39
barks, cleaning, 50
basal leaves, 33
baskets, 39
bee balm (*Monarda* spp.)
  bee balm salt recipe, 241
  general information, 34, 97, 160–163
  in herbal steam recipe, 227
  in wild rose honey recipe, 240
berberine, 157
Bidens alba. See Spanish needle (*Bidens alba*, *Bidens pilosa*, *Bidens frondosa*)
Bidens frondosa. See Spanish needle (*Bidens alba*, *Bidens pilosa*, *Bidens frondosa*)
Bidens pilosa. See Spanish needle (*Bidens alba*, *Bidens pilosa*, *Bidens frondosa*)
biennial plants, 27
bipinnate leaves, 32
bitters
  dandelion, 55, 56
  mugwort, 79
  yarrow, 119, 120
black walnut (*Juglans nigra*), 34, 48, 146–150
books, 246
botanical knowledge, 26
breastfeeding warning, wild lettuce (*Lactuca virosa*), 112
breast milk. See galactagogues
bulbs, 30

burdock (*Arctium lappa*)
   in decoction recipe, 213
   general information, 103–105

C

calculator, for tinctures, 217
calyces, 34, 47
calyx. *See* calyces
cardiovascular tonics
   kudzu, 89, 90
   motherwort, 123, 124
   reishi, 186, 187–188
carminatives
   bee balm, 161, 162
   garlic mustard, 75
   pine, 182
chaney root (*Smilax balbisiana*), 128
chickweed (*Stellaria media*)
   chickweed and wild greens pesto recipe, 242
   general information, 62–65
   in poultice recipe, 231
choloretics, dandelion, 55
circulatory stimulants, pine, 182
cleaning harvests, 48–50
cleavers (*Galium aparine*), 31, 58–61, 100
cold infusion
   general information, 143
   recipe, 211
community, 9–10
compound leaves, 32
cooling. *See* demulcents
coughing. *See* antitussives

D

dahlias, 30
dandelion (*Taraxacum officinale*), *12*, 22, 54–57

decoctions
   decoction recipe, 213
   general information, 207, 212
decongestants
   bee balm, 161, 162
   garlic mustard, 75, 76
   pine, 182, 183
dehydrators, 50, *51*
demulcents
   chickweed, 63, 64
   cleavers, 60
   honeysuckle, 165, 166
   linden, 191, 192
   mallow, 141, 142
   mullein, 95, 96
   plantain, 67, 68
   violet, 99, 100
diaphoretics
   elderberry, 136, 137–138
   linden, 191, 192
   motherwort, 123
   yarrow, 119, 120
diuretics
   burdock, 103, 104
   cleavers, 59
   dandelion, 55
   horsetail, 127, 128
   mallow, 141, 142
   Spanish needle, 115
   stinging nettle, 152, 153
   sumac, 173, 175
doctrine of signatures, 128
dosage
   cold infusions, 211
   decoctions, 213
   general information, 198
   glycerin extract, 223
   herbal vinegars, 225
   infusions, 209
   overnight infusions, 210

   tinctures, 219
dried plants, tincture calculator, 217
dropper bottles, 203
drug interactions, 196–197
drying harvests, 50–51

E

educational resources, online, 247
elderberry (*Sambucus canadensis*, *Sambucus nigra*, *Sambucus mexicana*)
   general information, 135–139
   in honeysuckle soda recipe, 244
elderflower. *See* elderberry (*Sambucus canadensis*, *Sambucus nigra*, *Sambucus mexicana*)
emmenagogues
   motherwort, 123, 124
   mugwort, 79, 82
endemic plants, 22
environmental variability, 27–28
Equisetum spp. *See* horsetail (*Equisetum* spp.)
essential oils, 229
   See also herbal oils
ethics in foraging, 16–21
expectorants
   elderberry, 136, 137–138
   mallow, 141, 142
   mullein, 95, 96

F

febrifuges, bee balm, 161
fevers. *See* febrifuges
field guides, 39

Index   249

flowers
    cleaning, 48–49
    general information, 31
    when to harvest, 47
foraging
    cleaning harvests, 48–50
    places to avoid, 43–44
    tools, 38–40
    when to forage, 46–48
    where to forage, 41–45
forested land, 43
freezing, 51
fruits
    general information, 34
    when to harvest, 48
funnels, 203

G

galactagogues, raspberry, 169, 170
Ganoderma lucidum. See reishi (*Ganoderma tsugae*, *Ganoderma lucidum*)
Ganoderma tsugae. See reishi (*Ganoderma tsugae*, *Ganoderma lucidum*)
garlic, wild, 30
garlic mustard (*Alliaria petiolata*)
    in bee balm salt recipe, 241
    general information, 27, 74–77
    in herbal vinegar recipe, 225
    in wild rose honey recipe, 240
ginger (*Zingiber officinale*), 29
glycerin, 201
glycerin extracts
    general information, 221
    glycerin extract recipe, 222–223

goldenrod (*Solidago* spp.), 41
goldenseal (*Hydrastis canadensis*), 157
greens, wild, 242

H

harvesting
    cleaning harvests, 48–50
    preserving harvests, 50–51
    when to harvest, 46–48
    See also specific plants
healing. See vulneraries
heart medications, and motherwort, 124
herbal hair wash
    general information, 229
    recipe, 235
herbal oils
    general information, 228–229
    recipe, 232–234
herbal steams
    general information, 226
    recipe, 227
herbal vinegars
    general information, 224
    recipe, 225
herbicide use, 41–42, 43–44
high traffic areas, 43–44
honey
    general information, 200, 238
    wild rose honey recipe, 239–240
honeysuckle (*Lonicera japonica*)
    general information, 31, 164–167
    in glycerin extract recipe, 223
    in herbal vinegar recipe, 225

honeysuckle soda recipe, 244
horsetail (*Equisetum* spp.)
    general information, 126–129
    in herbal hair wash recipe, 235
Hydrastis canadensis. See goldenseal (*Hydrastis canadensis*)
hyperaccumulators, 42
hypoglycemics, kudzu, 89, 90
hypotensives
    kudzu, 89, 90
    motherwort, 123, 124

I

identification books, 39
identifying plants
    general information, 27–28
    leaf identification, 32–33
    See also anatomy of plants; and specific plants
immunomodulators, reishi, 186, 187–188
immunostimulants, elderberry, 136, 137–138
infusions
    cold infusion recipe, 211
    general information, 206
    infusion recipe, 209
    making a strong infusion, 206–207
    overnight infusion recipe, 210
    storing, 208
inulin, 57, 104
invasive plants
    general information, 23
    honeysuckle, 164–167, 223, 225, 244

Japanese knotweed, *17*, 23, 29, *47*, 83–86, 219
kudzu, 23, 30, 44, 87–91
mimosa, *18*, 132, 177–180, 223, 240
Oregon grape, 156–159
Spanish needle, 114–117

J

Japanese honeysuckle. *See* honeysuckle (*Lonicera japonica*)
Japanese knotweed (*Polygonum cuspidatum*)
    general information, *17*, 23, 29, *47*, 83–86
    in tincture recipe, 219
jars, 39
Juglans nigra. *See* black walnut (*Juglans nigra*)

K

kitchen scales, 203
knives, 38–39, 203
kudzu (*Pueraria montana*)
    in decoction recipe, 213
    general information, 23, 30, 44, 87–91

L

labels, 203
Lactuca virosa. *See* wild lettuce (*Lactuca virosa*)
lanceolate leaves, 33
Laportea canadensis, 152
    See also stinging nettle (*Urtica dioica*)
leaf identification, 32–33
leaflets, 32
leaves
    cleaning, 48–49
    general information, 30–31
    when to harvest, 47
lenticels, 137
Leonurus cardiaca. *See* motherwort (*Leonurus cardiaca*)
lettuce, wild (*Lactuca virosa*), 41, 110–113
linden (*Tilia* spp.)
    in cold infusion recipe, 211
    general information, *42*, 132, 190–193
    in glycerin extract recipe, 223
    in honeysuckle soda recipe, 244
    in wild rose honey recipe, 240
lobed leaves, 33
Lonicera japonica. *See* honeysuckle (*Lonicera japonica*)
loupes, 40
lymphatics
    cleavers, 59, 60
    violet, 99, 100

M

Mahonia aquifolium. *See* Oregon grape (*Mahonia aquifolium*)
mallow (*Malva sylvestris*)
    in cold infusion recipe, 211
    general information, 141–143
Malva sylvestris. *See* mallow (*Malva sylvestris*)
mason jars, 202
medicinal foods
    bee balm salt recipe, 241
    chickweed and wild greens pesto recipe, 242
    general information, 238
    honeysuckle soda recipe, 244
    sumac lemonade recipe, 243
    wild rose honey recipe, 239–240
menstrua, 198–201
mimosa (*Albizia julibrissin*)
    general information, *18*, 132, 177–180
    in glycerin extract recipe, 223
    in wild rose honey recipe, 240
mixing bowls, 203
Monarda spp. *See* bee balm (*Monarda* spp.)
motherwort (*Leonurus cardiaca*)
    general information, 122–125, 132
    in tincture recipe, 219
mucilage
    linden, 192
    mallow, 141–143
    plantain, 68
    violet, 100
mugwort, 33
mugwort (*Artemisia vulgaris*)
    general information, 79–82
    in herbal oil recipe, 233
mullein (*Verbascum thapsus*)
    general information, 90, 95–97
    in herbal oil recipe, 234
    in infusion recipe, 209
musculoskeletal tonics, horsetail, 127, 128
mushrooms, cleaning, 50

N

native plants
　defined, 22
　vs. nonnative plants, 22–23
naturalized plants, 22–23
nature, connecting with, 10
nervines
　mimosa, 178
　motherwort, 123, 124
nettles, 11, 30
　See also stinging nettle (*Urtica dioica*)
nonnative plants, vs. native plants, 22–23
nutritives
　burdock, 103, 104
　chickweed, 63
　dandelion, 55
　horsetail, 127, 128
　plantain, 67, 68
　raspberry, 169, 170
　red clover, 107, 108
　Spanish needle, 115, 116
　stinging nettle, 152, 153
　sumac, 173, 175
　wild rose, 131, 133
nuts, cleaning, 50

O

oat (*Avena sativa*), 108
oil, 199
　See also essential oils; herbal oils
oneirogens, mugwort, 79, 81
one-third rule, 19, 21
onions, 30
opposite leaves, 33
Oregon grape (*Mahonia aquifolium*), 156–159

P

palmate leaves, 32
parks, 43
permission, asking for, 19–21
pesticide use, 41–42
petioles, 33
pine (*Pinus* spp.)
　general information, 181–184
　in herbal oil recipe, 234
　in herbal steam recipe, 227
　in herbal vinegar recipe, 225
　in wild rose honey recipe, 240
pinene, 183
pinnate leaves, 32
Plantago lanceolata. See plantain (*Plantago major, Plantago lanceolata*)
Plantago major. See plantain (*Plantago major, Plantago lanceolata*)
Plantago ovata, 68
　See also plantain (*Plantago major, Plantago lanceolata*)
plantain (*Plantago major, Plantago lanceolata*)
　general information, 22, 35, 66–69
　in herbal oil recipe, 234
　in poultice recipe, 231
plant anatomy, 28–35
plant ID
　general information, 27–28
　leaf identification, 32–33
　See also specific plants
plant knowledge, 26
plant medicine
　decoctions, 212–213
　general information, 196
　glycerin extracts, 221–223

herbal oils, 228–229, 232–234
herbal steams, 226–227
herbal vinegars, 224–225
infusions, 206–211
menstrua, 198–201
poultices, 228, 230–231
and pregnancy, 198
safety, 196–198
tinctures, 214–220
tools for making, 201–203
topical medicines, 228–235
poison sumac (*Toxicodendron vernix*), 174
　See also sumac (*Rhus typhina*)
Polygonum cuspidatum. See Japanese knotweed (*Polygonum cuspidatum*)
polypores, 187
potatoes, 30
pots, 201
poultices
　general information, 228
　poultice recipe, 230–231
prebiotics, burdock, 103, 104
pregnancy warnings
　herbal medicines and pregnancy, 198
　Japanese knotweed, 85
　motherwort, 124, 125
　mugwort, 82
　Oregon grape, 158
　sweet Annie, 73
　wild lettuce, 112
preserves, 43
preserving harvests, 50–51
presses, 202
pruners, 38–39
psyllium husk, 68

Pueraria montana. See kudzu
(*Pueraria montana*)

R

raspberry (*Rubus idaeus,*
Rubus strigosus)
general information, 168–171
in infusion recipe, 209
recipes
bee balm salt, 241
chickweed and wild greens
pesto, 242
cold infusion, 211
decoction, 213
glycerin extract, 222–223
herbal oil, 232–234
herbal steam, 227
herbal vinegar, 225
honeysuckle soda, 244
infusion, 209
overnight infusion, 210
poultice, 230–231
sumac lemonade, 243
tincture, 218–219
wild rose honey, 239–240
red clover (*Trifolium pratense*)
general information,
106–109
in herbal oil recipe, 234
in overnight infusion recipe,
210
reishi (*Ganoderma tsugae,*
Ganoderma lucidum)
in decoction recipe, 213
general information, 90,
185–189
residential areas, 41–42
resources, 246–247
respiratory tonics
mullein, 96
sweet Annie, 71, 72

responsible foraging, 17–21
See also ethics in foraging
resveratrol, 85
rhizomes, 29
Rhus typhina. See sumac (*Rhus typhina*)
risk status of plants, 18
roadsides, 43–45
roots
cleaning, 48–49
general information, 29
when to harvest, 46
Rosa spp. See wild rose (*Rosa* spp.)
rose, wild (*Rosa* spp.)
general information,
130–134
in honeysuckle soda recipe,
244
wild rose honey recipe,
239–240
rose hips, 47, 48
Rubus idaeus. See raspberry
(*Rubus idaeus,*
Rubus strigosus)
Rubus strigosus. See raspberry
(*Rubus idaeus, Rubus*
strigosus)

S

safety, 40, 196–198
Sambucus canadensis.
See elderberry
(*Sambucus canadensis,*
Sambucus nigra,
Sambucus mexicana)
Sambucus mexicana.
See elderberry
(*Sambucus canadensis,*
Sambucus nigra,
Sambucus mexicana)

Sambucus nigra. See elderberry
(*Sambucus canadensis,*
Sambucus nigra,
Sambucus mexicana)
scales, 203
scissors, 203
sedatives, wild lettuce, 111, 112
seeds
cleaning, 50
general information, 35
when to harvest, 48
Smilax balbisiana. See chaney
root (*Smilax balbisiana*)
Solidago spp. See goldenrod
(*Solidago* spp.)
Spanish needle (*Bidens alba,*
Bidens pilosa, Bidens
frondosa), 114–117
Stellaria media. See chickweed
(*Stellaria media*)
stems
cleaning, 48–49
general information, 30
when to harvest, 46–47
stewardship, 16–17, 21
See also ethics in foraging
stinging nettle (*Urtica dioica*)
general information, 151–155
in herbal hair wash recipe,
235
in overnight infusion recipe,
210
storage
of chickweed and wild greens
pesto, 242
of decoctions, 212, 213
glycerin extract, 223
of glycerin extracts, 223
of herbal hair wash, 235
of herbal oils, 233
of herbal vinegars, 225

Index 253

storage, continued
    of infusions, 208, 209, 210, 211
    of sumac lemonade, 243
    of tinctures, 219
    of wild rose honey, 239
strainers, 202
styptics, yarrow, 119, 120
sumac (*Rhus typhina*)
    general information, 172–176
    sumac lemonade recipe, 243
sweet Annie (*Artemisia annua*)
    general information, 70–73, 97
    in herbal steam recipe, 227
symptoms, 245

T

taproots, 29
Taraxacum officinale. See dandelion (*Taraxacum officinale*)
teas, 207
Tilia spp. See linden (*Tilia* spp.)
tinctures
    calculator, 217
    folk method, 214–215
    general information, 214
    ratios, 215–216
    technical method, 215–216
    tincture recipe, 218–219
    tips for making, 220
tools
    for foraging, 38–40
    for making plant medicines, 201–203
topical medicines
    general information, 228
    herbal hair wash, 229
    herbal oils, 228–229, 232–234
    poultices, 228, 230–231
Toxicodendron vernix. See poison sumac (*Toxicodendron vernix*)
transitional zones, 45
tricosane, 192
Trifolium pratense. See red clover (*Trifolium pratense*)
triterpenoids, 187
trowels, 40
tubers, 30

U

Urera baccifera, 152
    See also stinging nettle (*Urtica dioica*)
Urtica dioica. See stinging nettle (*Urtica dioica*)
urtication, 153
uterine tonics, raspberry, 169, 170

V

vegetable glycerin, 201
Verbascum thapsus. See mullein (*Verbascum thapsus*)
vinegar
    general information, 199–200
    herbal vinegars, 224–225
Viola odorata. See violet (*Viola odorata*, *Viola sororia*)
Viola sororia. See violet (*Viola odorata*, *Viola sororia*)
violet (*Viola odorata*, *Viola sororia*)
    general information, 98–101
    in herbal oil recipe, 233
volume, vs. weight, 215

vulneraries
    plantain, 67, 68
    yarrow, 119, 120

W

waste, avoiding, 19
water, 198–199
weight, vs. volume, 215
wellness tonics, stinging nettle (*Urtica dioica*), 152
whorled leaves, 32
wild garlic, 30
wild greens, 242
wild lettuce (*Lactuca virosa*), 41, 110–113
wild oregano. See bee balm (*Monarda* spp.)
wild rose (*Rosa* spp.)
    general information, 130–134
    in honeysuckle soda recipe, 244
    wild rose honey recipe, 239–240
    See also rose hips

Y

yarrow (*Achillea millefolium*)
    general information, 20–21, 119–121
    in herbal oil recipe, 234
    in infusion recipe, 209
    in poultice recipe, 231

Z

Zingiber officinale. See ginger (*Zingiber officinale*)

INTERIOR PHOTOGRAPHY CREDITS

© 13-Smile/iStock.com, 125; © 13Smile/Shutterstock.com, 212 l.; © 66squarefeet/Shutterstock.com, 86; © aga7ta/iStock.com, 96 t.; © alder7/iStock.com, 136; © Alena Vikhareva/iStock.com, 100; © Alex Manders/iStock.com, 162; © alexmak7/Shutterstock.com, 104 t.; © Alfredo Acero-Arevalo/Shutterstock.com, 178; © Alphotographic/iStock.com, 126; © Amelia/stock.adobe.com, 171; © Anna Nelidova/iStock.com, 156; © AnnaNel/Shutterstock.com, 12; Art Rachen/Unsplash, 194; © Arterra Picture Library/Alamy Stock Photo, 149 r.; © ArtZuka/Alamy Stock Photo, 123; © Avalon_Studio/iStock.com, 193; © Avis De Miranda/Shutterstock.com, 9; © avoferten/Shutterstock.com, 62–63, 242; © BambiG/iStock.com, 160; © Barbara Smits/Shutterstock.com, 241; © Bildagentur Zoonar GmbH/Shutterstock.com, 153; © blickwinkel/Alamy Stock Photo, 56 b., 112, 137 b.; © Brian Lasenby/Shutterstock.com, 181; © Bryan Reynolds/Alamy Stock Photo, 166 t.; © butterfly's dream/Shutterstock.com, 142 l.; © bykot photo/Shutterstock.com, 87; © c11yg/iStock.com, 6 r.; © Calin Tatu/Shutterstock.com, 164; © Chris Lawrence Images/Shutterstock.com, 97; © Christian Hutter/Alamy Stock Photo, 102; © ChWeiss/Shutterstock.com, 58, 191; © CMYK MAKER/Shutterstock.com, 174 b.; © Coppy/iStock.com, 141; © cristographic/stock.adobe.com, 163 t.; © dajingjing/Shutterstock.com, 70; © Dark_Side/Shutterstock.com, 190; Dmitry Makeev/CC BY-SA 4.0/Wikimedia Commons, 32 all but t.r., 33 all but b.l.; © Dr. Rainer Kerber/Shutterstock.com, 36; © Edita Medeina/Shutterstock.com, 138; © Ekaterina Senyutina/Alamy Stock Photo, 2; © Eletha15/Shutterstock.com, 52; © Emilio100/Shutterstock.com, 32 t.r.; © Equitano/Shutterstock.com, 99 b.; © Erkki Makkonen/Shutterstock.com, 55; © eugenehill/Shutterstock.com, 207; © FJAH/Shutterstock.com, 247; © Flower_Garden/Shutterstock.com, 24; © FotoHelin/Shutterstock.com, 234; © Francesca Leslie/Shutterstock.com, 161; © Frank Hecker/Alamy Stock Photo, 49, 77; © G_r_B/Shutterstock.com, 174 t.; © Gabriela Bertolini/Shutterstock.com, 72; © Galyna Syngaievska/Shutterstock.com, 29 t.; © Gerald Corsi/iStock.com, 99 t.; © Grigorii Pisotsckii/Shutterstock.com, 81; © gubernat/Shutterstock.com, 106; © Hamid Photography/iStock.com, 110; © haraldmuc/Shutterstock.com, 244; © Hecos/Shutterstock.com, 158 b.; © Heike Rau/Shutterstock.com, 159; © HJBC/iStock.com, 137 t.; © hjochen/Shutterstock.com, 76 l.; © homi/Shutterstock.com, 90; © hongquang09/iStock.com, 33 b.l.; © hsvrs/iStock.com, 31 b.; © ian600f/iStock.com, 84; © Ingrid Maasik/Shutterstock.com, 131; © Irina Zharkova/iStock.com, 96 b.; © istanbulimage/iStock.com, 173 t.; © lv-olga/Shutterstock.com, 149 l.; © jacquesvandinteren/iStock.com, 129; © James Aloysius Mahan V/Shutterstock.com, 185–186, 188; © James Nature Pics/Shutterstock.com, 179 r.; © Jana Krizova/Shutterstock.com, 121; © Jazmine/stock.adobe.com, 166 b.; © Jelena Gvozdenac Martinov/iStock.com, 120; © JIANG HONGYAN/Shutterstock.com, 30 b., 91; © JoannaTkaczuk/Shutterstock.com, 1, 31 t.; © John Ruberry/iStock.com, 7 l.; © Joseph Valencia/iStock.com, 165; © Jozef Gruszczyk/iStock.com, 83; © Julija Kumpinovica/Shutterstock.com, 128 l.; © Jun Zhang/iStock.com, 27, 74, 150; © Kabar/Shutterstock.com, 130; © Kajdi Szabolcs/iStock.com, 54; © Kaliwungu 73/Shutterstock.com, 128 r.; © kamuphoto/Shutterstock.com, 127; © KariHoglund/iStock.com, 5; © kariphoto/Shutterstock.com, 80 l.; © Kazakov Maksim/Shutterstock.com, 30 t.; K F/Unsplash, 118;

Interior photography credits, *continued*

© Kozioł Kamila/stock.adobe.com, 113; © Kristine Rad/Shutterstock.com, 170 r.; © Lapis2380/Shutterstock.com, 59; © LFRabanedo/stock.adobe.com, 95; © Lipatova Maryna/Shutterstock.com, 152, 155; © Lippert Photography/Shutterstock.com, 183 b.; © lixu/iStock.com, 14; © Liz Leyden/iStock.com, 85; © lubilub/iStock.com, 133 l.; © Lyudmila Lucienne/iStock.com, 111 b.; © lzf/Shutterstock.com, 64; © Madeleine Steinbach/Shutterstock.com, 56 t.; © Magdanatka/Shutterstock.com, 101; © magdasmith/iStock.com, 151; © Mantonature/iStock.com, 76 r.; © Marcus Harrison - plants/Alamy Stock Photo, 132; © Marek Mierzejewski/Shutterstock.com, 235; © marekuliasz/Shutterstock.com, 199 b.; © Marianne Pfeil/iStock.com, 34 t. ; © marineke thissen/Shutterstock.com, 209; © Marmalade Photos/Shutterstock.com, 45; Mars Vilaubi/© Storey Publishing, 7 r., 38, 51, 69, 173 b., 182, 183 t., 202, 204, 214, 219, 224, 240; © masa44/Shutterstock.com, 199 t.; © mdurajczyk/iStock.com, 17; © meunierd/Shutterstock.com, 184; © Michelle/stock.adobe.com, 239; © Miyuki Satake/Shutterstock.com, 105; © Nahhana/Shutterstock.com, 170 l., 233; © NANCY AYUMI KUNIHIRO/Shutterstock.com, 35; © Nattika/Shutterstock.com, 29 b.; © Nazaruk Nazar/Shutterstock.com, 243; © nblx/Shutterstock.com, 236; © Nick Pecker/Shutterstock.com, 172; © Nikolay Kurzenko/Shutterstock.com, 92; © nnattalli/Shutterstock.com, 11, 167, 177, 221; © Nurdeana Cahyaningrum/Shutterstock.com, 116; © ok_fotoday/Shutterstock.com, 34 b.; © Oleg Kovtun/iStock.com, 158 t.; © Oleg Marchak/iStock.com, 67; © Oli S photography/Shutterstock.com, 47 r.; © olko1975/Shutterstock.com, 60 b., 104 b.; © Orest Lyzhechka/Shutterstock.com, 20, 65, 71, 75, 78, 80 r.;

124, 226; © PaniYani/Shutterstock.com, 168; © Pedro1987/Shutterstock.com, 180; © Peter Turner Photography/Shutterstock.com, 147; © petrovichlili/Shutterstock.com, 144; © PFM photostock/Shutterstock.com, 169; © Photo digitaal.nl/Shutterstock.com, 192; © piemags/nature/Alamy Stock Photo, 111 c.; © piemags/nature/Alamy Stock Photo, 187; © Pilar Picas/Shutterstock.com, 142 r.; © Primi2/Shutterstock.com, 18; © Reikara/Shutterstock.com, 197; © Rex May/Alamy Stock Photo, 122; © Richard Becker/Alamy Stock Photo, 94; © rustamank/Shutterstock.com, 98; © Sandra Burm/Shutterstock.com, 23; © sasirin pamai/iStock.com, 212 r.; © Scalia Media/Shutterstock.com, 44; © seven75/iStock.com, 66; © shalom3/Shutterstock.com, 175; © shepherdsatellite/Shutterstock.com, 107; © simona pavan/Shutterstock.com, 114; © sisi2017/Shutterstock.com, 223; © skhoward/iStock.com, 163 b.; © Soeren Schulz/Shutterstock.com, 157; © spline_x/Shutterstock.com, 109; © STUDIO75/Alamy Stock Photo, 146; © tamu1500/Shutterstock.com, 89; © Tatiana Belkina/Shutterstock.com, 22; © temmuzcan/Shutterstock.com, 6 l.; © This_is_JiHun_Lee/Shutterstock.com, 26, 115; © Tim Mainiero/Shutterstock.com, 88; © Tom Meaker/iStock.com, 60 t.; © Tom Meaker/Shutterstock.com, 140; © Tomas Vynikal/Shutterstock.com, 47 l.; © undefined undefined/iStock.com, 111 t.; © UntitledR/Shutterstock.com, 231; © Valeriy Shevtsov/iStock.com, 108; © Varga Jozsef Zoltan/Shutterstock.com, 148; © wepix/iStock.com, 135; © xpixel/Shutterstock.com, 68; Yuri Antonenko/Unsplash, 133 r.; © zhongguo/iStock.com, 179 l.; © Zoonar GmbH/Alamy Stock Photo, 42; © ZoranKrstic/Shutterstock.com, 210